Book Title:

Dr. AI - A New Precedent in US Healthcare

Authored by Mohamed Tanana

LLM, MHA, MA, MCIArb

FOREWORD

Fascinated by technology and its inclusion in health sciences and management, I was intrigued by the works of Kim and Song (2020) in *Technology and Health: Promoting Attitude and Behavior Change.* Around the time, I was interested in the possibilities of artificial intelligence in health management and sciences. By taking notes of the health issues in the existing paradigm of healthcare in the U.S., I obliged to answer them through usage of technology in my mind; and later, decided to incorporate that in a book. Having first-hand experience on the issues of healthcare, its increasing quality gap with issues faced by practitioners and patients; I was able to stay motivated throughout the course of writing this book.

The inclusion of work experience in the U.S. healthcare enabled me to incorporate existing issues in health sector while I focused myself reading through technological breakthroughs elsewhere in the world that optimized health sector performance. National Health Services (NHS) UK has a comprehensive and centralized health system that monitors standardized healthcare practice while ensuring that the patient receive optimal care quality. In the U.S. the presence of privatized institution intrigued me towards the betterment of healthcare system through technology. Works of Genetika+, HealthXL and other tools using predictive analysis motivated my book further to elaborate on the expertise and advantages of technology in healthcare sector. We believe that technology is an additional, yet a very competitive participant of quality healthcare betterment.

In these chapters, you will find introduction to technology in healthcare, contribution of technology to improve practitioners' delivery of quality and technological contribution of AI in assisting patients to control the workload of US healthcare mechanism. It is my hope that this book will provide healthcare providers and researchers, with new knowledge, skills and insights, as well as guidance and solutions to medical errors and to help narrow the quality gap within the organizational workplace. Further, it is my hope to inspire healthcare practitioners to take action that will improve on healthcare needs of their providers, and bring positive change in the lives of their patients and loved ones. Moreover, the book offers healthcare providers and practitioners, as well as researchers, a path to organizational and systemic growth, mindfulness, self-discovery and improvement, and transformational development within the healthcare system.

I am hoping that the reader will find value and inspiration in this book.

PREFACE

The book is focused on the escalating healthcare issues in the US and the inclusion of technology to respond to the quality gap. Motivated by working in the healthcare industry, I had the opportunity to explore the issues faced by practitioners and the challenges they adhere in day-to-day work engagement. Technology answered complications to healthcare complexities including research, practice and management. Having a stream of knowledge in both domains which are healthcare and technology; I was inclined towards penning down the improvements that can be made in bridging healthcare quality gaps in the industry. Dr. AI is originally focused on the inclusion of AI in closing the quality gap in healthcare to improve effectiveness of healthcare sector in the US. My experience in assisting patients through the best possible outcomes from health management has enabled me to understand the importance of artificial intelligence in the current world.

ACKNOWLEDGEMENTS

The book is based on the key findings and health data collected by US department of healthcare (National Institutes of Health) and the publishing sources that assisted in finding the right technologies to address health issues in the existing world. Therefore, the author acknowledges the support of publishing sources such as *BMJ Open, Frontiers in Digital Health, Health policy and technology, BMC health services research, Healthcare Informatics Research* and *Technology in Society* among several other. It provided the book with key insights on the development of artificial intelligence and enabled the author to address key issues in US healthcare system.

I would like to thank my family for their immense support during the time I have dedicated to this book and their understanding of my commitment to improve healthcare mechanism in the US. Their unwavering love, attention, encouragement and understanding assisted me to allocate desired time and attention to the book. My beloved wife, Alissar, whose constant support enabled me to extend my attention towards the subject. And also my children Zahra, Zainab, Mahdi, and Zachariah for their patience. I must also extend my appreciation to my sister Fatme for her unwavering inspiration and motivation. My friends also deserve an acknowledgement who motivated me every step of the way to pen down the breakthroughs of technology in healthcare sector.

My mentor guided me through the key concepts that I should discuss in the book. With his expertise, I was able to navigate through complexities in technology and write in a way that is understandable for the readers and they acknowledge the importance of technology in modern healthcare. His constructive feedback enabled me to revisit my initial draft to improve my book writing style and provide meticulous attention to detail for enhanced effectiveness.

Also, I would like to thank my publisher, for believing in the project and assisting me in spreading the importance of technology in modern healthcare in the US. The key editorial insights and dedication elevated the quality of this manuscript, and for creating a captivating cover that truly captures the essence of the book. Lastly, but not the least, I would acknowledge and oblige to the support of this book's reader whose unwavering interest motivate authors like me to delve into the complexities of technology and their importance in improving our daily lives. Your interest and curiosity are what make this journey worthwhile.

List of Abbreviations

AI – Artificial Intelligence

AR – Augmented Reality

CDS – Clinical Decision System

CNN – Convolution Neural Network

DCR – Digital Clock and Recall

DL – Deep Learning

EHR – Electronic Health Record

EKG – Electrocardiogram

EMR – Electronic Medical Record

FWA – Fraud, Waste and Abuse detection and prevention

GDP – Gross Domestic Product

HIPPA – Health Insurance Portability and Accountability Act

HRIS – Human Resource Information System

IOM – American Institute of Medicine

IT – Information Technology

MECC – Making Every Contact Count

ML – Machine Learning

NLP – Natural Language Processing

PPACA – Patient Protection and Affordable Care Act

SVM – Support Vector Machine

TAM – Technology Acceptance Model

US – United States

Table of Contents

List of Figures

List of Tables

Chapter 1:

Healthcare and Need for Technology

AI promised a new norm of enhanced healthcare in the US. In 2018, there was a 290% increase in spending on United States (US) healthcare despite the increasing quality gaps in the region (compared to 1980) (American Medical Association, 2023). Increased access to healthcare, controlled administrative burden, and investment in primary care were primarily reported to increase healthcare efficiency of a region. Currently, the US healthcare system is accused of not removing cost barriers for efficient healthcare which challenges accessibility of patients. However, through appropriate usage of technology, accessibility of patient care can be significantly enhanced.

Furthermore, there is a negligence of universal healthcare system which increases patient spending on healthcare accounting for 16.9% of their gross domestic product (GDP) in 2019 (Rama, 2019). Technology was accounted as a methodology to control administrative burden within the healthcare sector. Inclusion of information based decision making on patient arrival, level of incentive care, and patient satisfaction monitored with technology enhanced the level of decision making along with increased efficiency of healthcare (Amann et al., 2020).

Involvement of negligence in diagnostics, surgery and treatment were covered in malpractice in healthcare sector. Malpractice is a commonly discussed phenomenon in healthcare sector with respect to its management. However, malpractice involved a range of medical activities which are overlooked by healthcare professional yet they go unreported. The following figure 1 showed medical errors made by healthcare professional in terms of diagnostics, treatments and operations. Since complications range from minor to fatal, they often go unreported as health complications or side-effects of healthcare for patient.

Therefore, there was an increased need of technology which prioritized patient's interest and account for negligence of healthcare professionals (Soroya et al., 2021). Currently, $40 million investment has been made spent on development of information technology (IT) and implementation for healthcare sector in the US (Vega and Kizer, 2020). The increased investment on technology was thoroughly motivated to improve patient care and minimize quality gaps through identification of negligence of professionals and categorization of health complications occurred in patients.

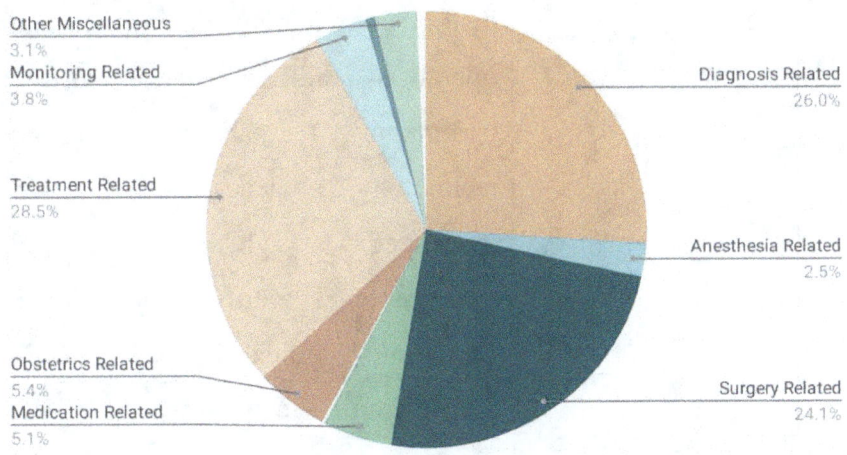

Figure 1 Causes of Medical Malpractice Claims (Gobel, 2022)

Technology has a proven impact on improvement of healthcare through efficient replacement mechanism of human resources. Traditionally, human resources incorporated their decision based on their limited processing capacity of abundant information. However, through technology (and big data analysis), computer based decision making has marginalized patient waiting time, enhanced experience of healthcare visits and controlled the quality gap within the dynamics of healthcare sector in the US. The following table 1 showed some of the commonly reported advantages of technology in healthcare:

Table 1 Benefits of Technology in Healthcare

Benefits of Technology in Healthcare	
Access to medical records	Patient's medical records and their history of treatment, diagnostics and operations readily assisted in existing treatment of patients. Through technology, accessibility was trivialized which ensured enhancement of healthcare. Electronic Medical Records (EMR) or Electronic Health Records (EHR) were readily utilized for technological access (Murala et al., 2023).
Marginalized medical errors	American Institute of Medicine (IOM) reported 98,000 deaths annually occur due to medical errors and malpractice. Clinical Decision System (CDS) provides safety information for practitioners which marginalizes medical errors within practice.
Increased patient care	Traditionally, results of blood pressure, blood glucose level and

	other foundational test were only provided to patients; however, with increased technology, institutions are able to store their test results in digital format for increased accessibility and transparency for future treatment of patients.
Enhanced patient education	Increased use of PatientPoint and Digital Health Coalition by US physicians has showed an increased use of technology in healthcare. 75% of the physicians believe that increment in patient education can lead them to being extensively satisfied with their healthcare experience in the US (PatientPoint, 2023).
Reduction in cost	Medical errors in US hospitals occurs costs over $20 billion annually. Through medical EMR, outpatient care cost can be reduced by 3% (El Khatib et al., 2022). Furthermore, a cloud powered medical EMR can empower the entire industry to treat a

	specific patient anywhere around the country which enhances the overall quality level while controlling cost of operations.

Malpractice in US is often defended by claims made by practitioners of unavailability of information or inaccuracy of the patient condition as reported by the patients (Schacht et al., 2022). The inclination of the practitioners as per the '*good medical practice*' includes making informed decisions. However, 33% of malpractice claims result of misdiagnosis errors in the US which has alarmed the health sector (Figure 2). The awareness of patients regarding their illnesses and conditions in the US has significantly increased after news channels have participated in exposing brutal realities of medical practice.

Therefore, there was an increased need of technology to improve and improvise the existing medical practice. It could be achieved by incorporating technology to access EMR or EHR for patient health's record. Usage of technology in healthcare sector was inclined towards assistance in surgery; however, the requirement was rather largely focused towards management. Practitioners reported that patients were not able to efficiently describe their medical conditions which led to misdiagnosis (Murala et al., 2023). Contrarily, through technology, medical information accessed from EMR and EHR can readily enhance the level of effectiveness of diagnosis.

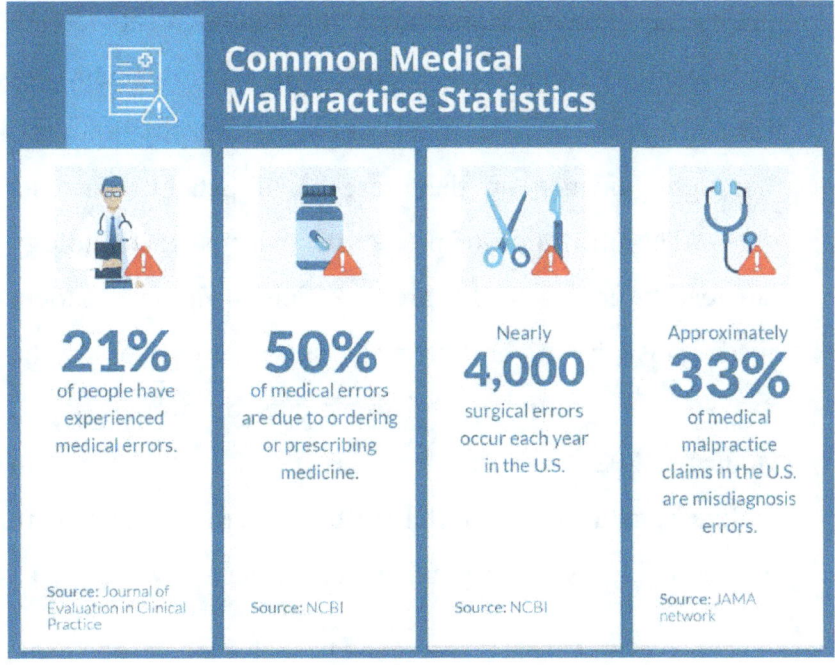

Figure 2 Malpractice Claims in the US (Dimetman, 2022)

By profession, it was noticed that physicians were accused of malpractice more commonly than the rest of specialized practitioners (Figure 3). 33% of the physicians spent more than 40 hours defending lawsuits which led to compromised productivity on their end to enhance their healthcare practices (Bookman and Zane, 2020). Furthermore, it was noticed that the increased time spent on the lawsuits readily marginalized their ability to control the quality gap in patient care.

Therefore, inclusion of technology was the only precedent left to incorporate in healthcare to marginalize quality gap. Patient expectations and treatment satisfaction significantly increased through the involvement of technology as it presented unbiased information and thorough guidance on the presence of patient's disease.

The utilization of predictive analysis in technology can readily enable healthcare to efficiently reduce patient misdiagnosis by a significant margin while controlling the cost spent on surgeries and treatments by 50% (Foresee Medical, 2023). Therefore, usage of technology in healthcare is a vital requirement of modernized healthcare system in the US to marginalize quality gap.

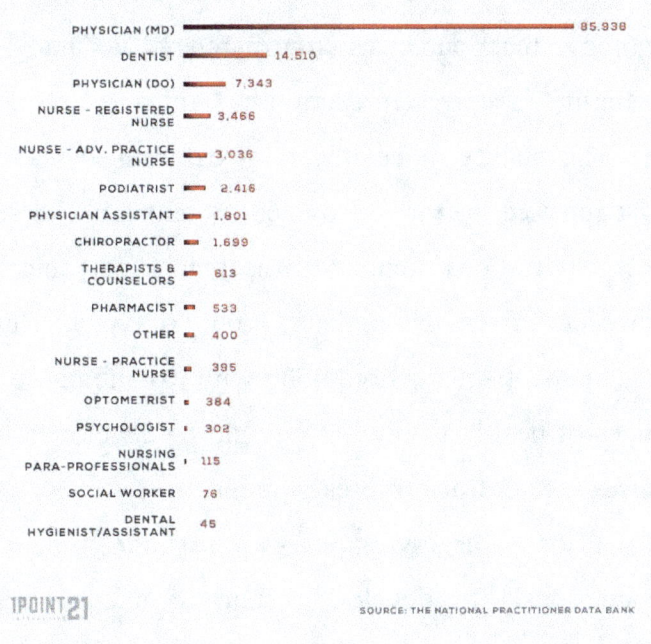

Figure 3 Malpractice Reports by Profession (Rosenbaum, 2019)

The 5.1% of patients' death was caused by medicine related errors which primarily constituted of errors from pharmacists or diagnostician who misinterpreted patient's disease and prescribed a different medicine (Figure 1; Rodziewicz, 2020). In case of US, the rising number of claims over maligned prescriptions and ineffectiveness of drugs have significantly increased and healthcare laws have instructed pharmacist as a channel of second opinion to doctor's prescription. However, pharmacist do not have the expertise of being an authenticated diagnostician which leads to persistence of medical errors. Therefore, there was an increased need of technology that enhances transparency, accuracy, and accessibility of correct prescription (Akhtar et al., 2020).

The quality of healthcare is determined by patient satisfaction with services provided by entire health sector; unmet expectations generates discontent for the entire health sector from the patient's point of view. Thus, to enhance patient satisfaction along with expanding on good practices of health, technology should be developed which enhances the accuracy of prescriptions.

Prior to surgery, patients are required to be treated with anesthesia to develop a state of unconsciousness which assists a surgeon in completing their surgeries effectively (Ahn et al., 2019). However, in accordance to figure 1, it was noticed that patients' death in the US through anesthesia account for 2.5% of the total death rate (Gobel, 2022). Primarily, anesthesia related deaths are caused by circulatory failure due to hypovolemia along with over-dosage of agents including hiopentone, opioids, or benzodiazepines (Manougian and Zangbar, 2022). Thus, there is an increased need of technology which studies the immunity of body to anesthetic agents along with the required dosage to be calculated by technology. Human calculations on dosage can lead to significant errors.

However, through EHR, patient's health record can be transparently accessed to determine their level of immunity and body condition to withstand anesthetic agents. Contrarily, the chances of human error persist within the range of 30% to 40%. Furthermore, AI based technology can assist anesthesiologist to control anesthetic drug in human body to avoid laryngospasm and subsequent oxygenation issues (McKendrick et al., 2021).

In the US, $2.5 trillion of its GDP in spent on healthcare which constitutes of 17.2% of GDP of US (Surkunte, 2022). The healthcare expenses have increased at a faster rate than inflation which has significantly enhanced the need of technology in healthcare. However, there are a range of reasons which resist the implementation of technology in healthcare that includes:

1. Imperceptive adoption of technology in healthcare
2. Increased cost of technology
3. Consumer price sensitivity
4. Limited incentive for health practitioners
5. Overutilization of technology

6. Lack of advancements in chronic disease prevention

7. Defensive medical costs

US has always been prudent on enhancing their healthcare sector with advancements in technology while increasing restrictive barriers for healthcare practitioners which includes litigation in malpractice cases, imposition of fines and termination of license. However, it was determined that such restrictive barriers readily enhance the level of technological expertise required as practitioners are adamant on prescribing extra tests and medicines to ensure that patient fully recovers which is an added cost to the government (Benitez et al., 2020). Therefore, incorporation of technology can readily provide a doctor with a second opinion on comprehensive examination of patient body while giving an insight to the physicians regarding patient's health concerns.

There is an inability of patients in reining their respective physicians to the complications they face (Tariq et al., 2020). Physicians are required to test their complications through laboratory while incorporating uncertainties on patient's communicational errors. Furthermore, poor documentation of critical information by practitioners is also among the contributors of quality gap in healthcare. Therefore, technological expertise was required to effectively record physician and patient's communication in a method which could be easily followed by patients. The emphasis of patient care is on following instruction of physicians while being critical of treatment methods they prescribed to follow. Otherwise, criticality of patient's complications may increase and could result in malpractice. Thus, technological intervention can lead as a reminder for the patient to follow physician's instruction while trivializing the information for patients to readily understand (Wurcel et al., 2019). The preceding process can significantly bridge the quality gap in existing healthcare system in the US. However, technologies were being reined into healthcare sector; yet the rate was slower than what was desired in improving quality of healthcare in the US.

Healthcare practitioners have increasingly collaborated to the collection of data which can empower implementation of technology in the industry (Awad et al., 2021). However, the willingness, determination and financial constraints are yet to be addressed in healthcare industry. In line with financial requirements, 40% of the US healthcare providers have noticed an increase in their technological budget (Surkunte, 2022).

Furthermore, federal government has introduced significant reforms amidst the increased need of technology in healthcare sector including the Health Insurance Portability and Accountability Act (HIPPA) of $19.2 billion to be invested in data management. The Patient Protection and Affordable Care Act (PPACA) ensured that healthcare practitioners readily emphasize on marginalizing the cost of treatments for patients. However, the resistance occurred in malpractice where marginalization of treatment may increase the quality gap in healthcare. Therefore, practitioners readily defended their approach through incorporation of various testing services prior to beginning of treatment. Such measures have extensively increased the need of technology in US healthcare that can optimize the process in healthcare while closing in on the quality gap.

PPACA was primarily designed to enhance affordability of healthcare across US through premium tax credits (Stone and Hoffman, 2010). However, the increased budget on health care spending was a pressing issue for the government. Therefore, there was an increased need of technology to optimize the operations of healthcare which bridges quality gap while enhancing the derivatives of practitioner outcomes towards their respective patients. The inclination of technology in healthcare has sufficiently enhanced the usage of *"making every contact count"* (MECC) (Phillips, 2019). Conventional practices primarily neglected health complications which did not show rigorous sign of development or toll on human body. However, with incorporation of technology, practitioners have embraced the usage of MECC which enables them to test patient's likelihood to develop diseases or non-active complication in their body to bridge quality gap. Contrarily, PPACA also covered the enhanced cost of technology in health framework which provided a legislation on technological improvement for sustenance of hospitals. Therefore, the role of government was found to be critical in terms of implementation of technology in health care.

Chapter 2:

AI in Healthcare Management

Artificial Intelligence (AI) in healthcare management has ensured that the inclusion of quality management is prioritized. The embracement of AI in healthcare management has marginalize time taken for clinicians to manage their time for patient management. AI has further contributed to automate tasks which require controlled analytical and human interaction. Moreover, the usage of AI has enhanced diagnostic levels by providing second opinions to consultants using the patient history.

Since AI readily trains itself as per patient information, its decision making significantly improves which controls the margin of error for practitioners. The usage of AI has further incentivized data management; human intelligence to aid recruitment, selection and management; remote surgery; drug discovery and clinical trial design (Panch et al., 2019). Each of the preceding aspect has contributed towards marginalized quality gaps as human resources in forms of health practitioners often neglected critical details which proved to be fatal for patients. Therefore, incorporation of AI has readily facilitated healthcare in terms of efficient management of information and patient treatment. Figure 4 showed some of the common benefits of AI in healthcare.

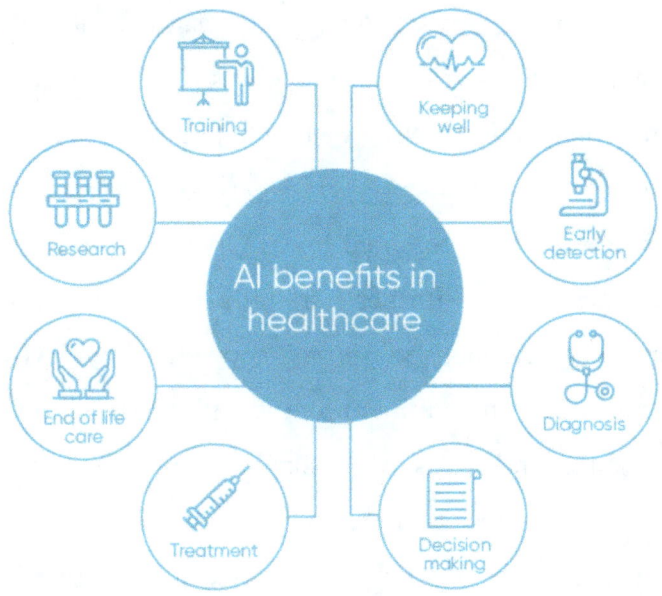

Figure 4 AI Benefits in Healthcare (Willink, 2021)

The alignment of practitioners to provide better healthcare can occur through extensive accountability. However, marginalized management experience of healthcare professional does not readily fuel the inclusion of performance management. Through AI, human resource management system (HRIS) and machine learning (ML), performance management can thoroughly be automated which monitors performance and satisfaction index of practitioners in an unbiased manner (Morley et al., 2020).

Traditionally, patient survey was utilized to evaluate performance of practitioners; however, with discrepancies in their behavior, it was discredited as an optimal source of practitioner performance. Through AI, and data on their performance such as time taken to see a patient, visits undertaken to complete treatment and overall patient experience; a collaborative report on practitioner performance can be obtained from AI which empowers the management for further training of practitioners. Contrarily, personalized portal powered by AI can efficiently recommend practitioners with feedback on their performance and areas of weakness they should readily consider for increased efficiency.

Treatment related malpractice was the primary contributor of increased quality gaps in the US. However, inclusion of second opinion can sufficiently improve diagnostic accuracy by providing a distinct point of view to patient's condition. Contrarily, for all treatments and increased demand of healthcare, usage of second opinion was a lengthy process adding to the complexities of healthcare management (Kompa et al., 2021). In case of AI, it was observed as a scientific and academic provider of second opinion solely based on facts providing unbiased solution or interpretation of patient's conditions. Therefore, a patient database management powered by AI can significantly marginalize quality gap within the healthcare sector of the US. Contrarily, diagnosis was observed to contribute to 26% of malpractice statistics in the US (Figure 1).

With embracement of AI, diagnostics can be sufficiently improved with efficient data management of patient history. It is important to realize that the malpractice in diagnostic occurs due to extensive presence of patient history present with practitioners and consultant that they fail to interpret existing condition of the patient. Thus, through AI, an unbiased diagnostic opinion can be formulated to control the quality gap in healthcare.

AI in healthcare research has significantly improved health outcomes and patient experiences (Lee and Yoon, 2021). Clinical decision support tools have enhanced decisions on treatments, medication and mental health needs of patients. AI has further benefitted the area of medical imaging where it analyses CT-scans, X-rays, MRIs and other technologically empowered tests by providing insights that a radiologist may neglect. It empowers practitioners to pursue informed decisions as per 'good medical practice' which controls the rate of misdiagnosis in clinical decisions (Bontemps-Hommen et al., 2019). It was noticed that the inclusion of technology in modern medical practice has significantly marginalized malpractice reports (Figure 4). However, there is a significant ratio of malpractice reports which has to be addressed through the inclusion of AI in healthcare management. $38.5 billion have been paid out to victims of medical malpractice (Cha, 2021).

Assuming a $400,000 annual salary of a radiologist performing redundant task, an automation in the field of radiology in conducting tests and handling reports can save significant capital of the healthcare industry to treat their patient while enhancing quality through automation. Moreover, it can enable the healthcare industry to transfer the benefit of affordable healthcare to the patient's as well. In the US, majority of the patients have raised their voices against the burdening prices of healthcare in the country (Kompa et al., 2021).

However, the inclusion of research and development has also been the part of medical cost incurred by patients. As a result, the modern healthcare system requires extensive efforts from technological industry to provide result oriented solution to bridge quality gaps in the healthcare industry. Furthermore, the augmented reality

(AR) programs have also intensified the effectiveness of training programs and research for practitioners enabling them to treat the patient with effective experience through AR.

In addition to the $38.5 billion spent on victims of malpractice, and additional amount of $29 billion is spent on documentation errors annually which are preventable. Contrarily, the number has doubled since the incorporation of technology primarily due to lack of technology acceptance in healthcare sector which is enhanced with limited technological expertise among healthcare practitioners.

Therefore, inclusion of AI in healthcare can significantly control the human intervention required to maintain EHR and EMR. AI can be incorporated to efficiently maintain patient's health record constituting of their entire healthcare journey. Thus, it was important that clinical strategies were adjusted to overcome the high payments in terms of medical malpractice.

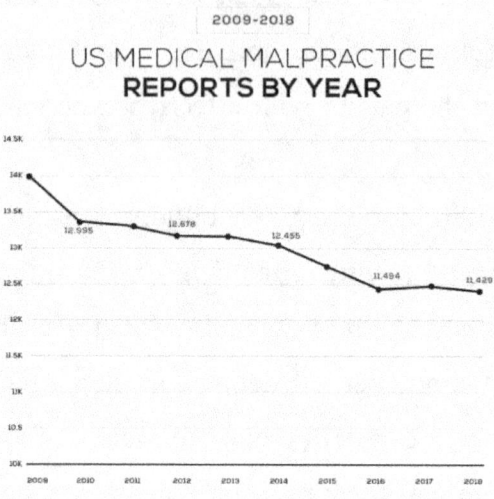

Figure 5 US Medical Malpractice Reports by Year (Rosenbaum, 2019)

The provision of AI in healthcare management is limitless. However, the implementation strategies of AI are extensively scattered which proves to be a complication for adaptation in modern healthcare system (El-Gazzar and Stendal, 2020). However, it was determined that the readiness of healthcare amidst modernization is a beneficial time for AI to be incorporated in healthcare management. Management errors are often neglected in treating a patient based on their criticality and there are increased number of arguments to offset management error complains. Contrarily, incorporation of technology has readily enabled hospitals and institutions to marginalize management errors. Incorporation of AI can significantly optimize healthcare management performance by eliminating biasness from decision making. The following are fundamental advantages of incorporating AI in healthcare management:

- Enhance evidence based practices by decision support system
- Advise on tailored clinical research trials
- Real-time diagnosis for efficient decision making

The aforementioned advantages enhance the proficiency level of healthcare management in pursuit to bridge the quality gap. However, implementation of AI in the sector can be met by resistance to change management in accordance to technology acceptance model (TAM) (Kamal et al., 2020). Therefore, it is recommended that the process of implementation is set according to the expertise of practitioner where they observe AI as a facilitator in bridging quality and not as a complication in their existing process of treatment and management of patients.

Machine Learning (ML) has been a key development for AI in healthcare management. International Business Machine Corporation (IBM)'s Watson AI system has incorporated the use of ML to readily process patient information against the existing data set to make predictions about the outcomes of the treatment which has readily increased the accuracy of patient treatment, and diagnosis (Strickland, 2019). Data science has readily been incorporated in ML for extensive detail oriented work on treatment framework and probabilities of successful treatment (Strickland, 2019).

The unnoticeable diseases in a patient can be readily interpreted through data analysis techniques which can compare patient's condition with symptoms of other patients through presence of EMR and EHR and it can assist practitioners in enhancing their quality of practice. Furthermore, Natural Language Processing (NLP) is among the latest development of AI in healthcare and it has enabled clinical documentation, clinical decision support, dictation and EMR implications along with review management and sentiment analysis. The following figure shows some of the common features of NLP that healthcare incorporates.

Since there is a limited technological expertise among health practitioners in understanding fundamentals of AI while the technological experts are not sound with needs of health care sector; NLP, as a program, integrates machine learning for technologically inexperienced individuals which leads to significant development in technological advancements in healthcare (Hasikin et al., 2023). In technical terms, NLP uses unstructured information in trivial formats for physicians to incorporate decision making. Its ability to comprehend human speech and implement it in machine learning tool has readily advanced its implementation in healthcare sector. NLP has enabled physicians to incorporate information for better decision making and analytics of patient's health cycle prior to generation of prescription. Primarily, NLP readily sorts unstructured data by mapping essential concepts and values which empowers physicians to empower decision making through knowledge management (Xia et al., 2022). Some of the common advantages of NLP includes the following:

Table 2 Advantages of NLP

Clinical Documentation	Speech Recognition
Computer Assisted Coding	Data Mining Research
Automated Registry Reporting	Clinical Decision Support
Clinical Trial Matching	Prior Authorization
AI Chatbots and Virtual Scribe	Hierarchal Condition Categories
Dictation and EMR Implications	Root Cause Analysis

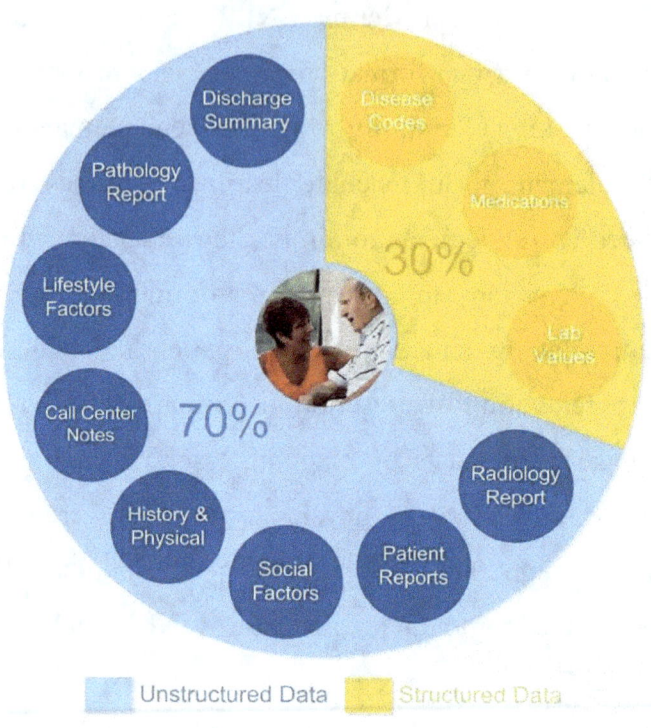

*Figure 6 Usage of NLP in Healthcare through Structured and Unstructured
Data (AltexSoft, 2021)*

NLP can be incorporated in health care industry to increase patient health awareness, improve quality of care provided by practitioners by better decision making, improve patient interaction with healthcare provider and EHR along with identification of patient's critical care needs (Xia et al., 2022). Furthermore, predictive analysis in diagnostic process by NLP can assist healthcare sector in identification of high-risk patients who highly contribute to the death rates in US. Thus, incorporation of technologies such as NLP in IBM Watson, Isabel and MXModal are extensively empowered with the usage of NLP. It enables the healthcare technological providers to have an interactive user interface which can be conveniently used by health practitioners despite their controlled exposure to technological tools. Moreover, it can also significantly contribute to catalyze the process of implementation of technology in healthcare sector and address resistance in change management. NLP also offers to streamline workflow without incorporating the usage of micromanagement in the field of healthcare through implementation of technology in accordance to the need of medical facility.

AI can only be implemented in healthcare with efficiency of data available to train AI model (Chen and Decary, 2020). It was determined that the extensive nature of data can enable AI to make efficient decision based on prior outcomes which can contribute to abridgement of quality gap in US healthcare. However, the data collection can only be empowered through incorporation of technology. Thus, companies like Deloitte are increasingly contributing to research of healthcare data collection through cloud computing and solutions (Deloitte, 2023).

The company stated that cloud computing traditional benefits include ability to optimize cost, scalability and flexibility. However, the modern researches revealed that the achievement is persistent in creating patient centric intervention in healthcare (El-Gazzar and Stendal, 2020; Strickland, 2019).

Therefore, incorporation of cloud computing in healthcare can sufficiently enhance the level of quality provided in healthcare management. Furthermore, the accessibility of data can empower all hospitals and institutions to use collected data for better decision making. It was noticed that the management lapse was persistent due to lack of information or lack of experience of decision maker. However, through cloud technologies, and AI, managers can readily improve their decision making in prioritizing patient's need and requirement (Xia et al., 2022).

Amidst the increasing need of testing services and false alarms for tests, Iterative Health has made a breakthrough research in gastroenterology department which incorporates computational algorithms that leads to identification of patients who are eligible for testing of inflammatory bowel disease. Incorporation of such technologies have readily marginalized testing requirements in modern healthcare framework.

In case of Iterative Health, it has trivialized information processing and detection through in camera view where a bounding box appears when it detects an anomaly in bowel system of a human (Iterative Health, 2023). Through the appearance of bounding box, healthcare management can take its desired action to treat the patient and determine their level of urgency. The transparency provided by Iterative Health in modern healthcare framework is set to improve detection of bowel diseases along with treatment methods. However, such technologies are needed for all organs of human body. Thus, there is an increased emphasis on the usage of AI in healthcare management to optimize the process.

Babylon Health is an AI powered applications which aims to be a virtual health assistant for patients. The application was designed to marginalize traffic in hospital and other health institutions. It was noticed that patients were extensively misinformed about diagnosis of their disease through reading blogs on online platforms (DeBord et al., 2018). However, through the usage of AI powered technologies, patients could rapidly identify root cause of their problem while knowing the right consultant for their problem.

The application has significantly marginalized unwanted hospital visits from patient's end while extensively enabling practitioners to focus on urgent medical attention. Following figure showed the help seeking feature of Babylon Health app which was primarily designed to automatically address patients need. Such technologies have reinstated patient's and population's belief on modernized healthcare system. Integration of technology in healthcare has comprehensively improved health framework in the US yet the cost of implementation is found to be high amidst technology boom in the current market conditions.

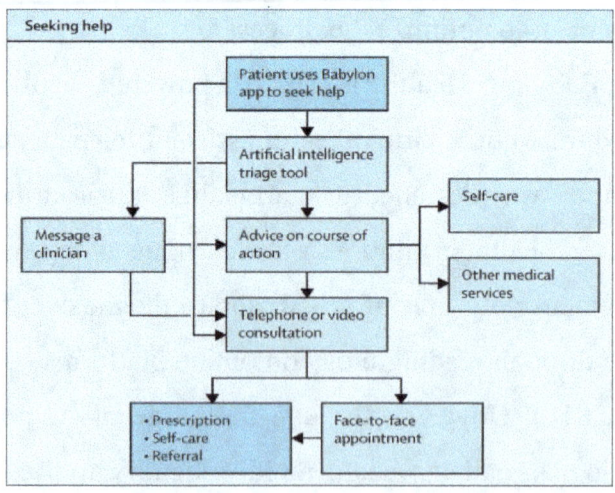

Figure 7 Babylon Application Workflow (Burki, 2019)

Chapter 3

Contribution of AI in Healthcare for Practitioners

L inus health is among the recent breakthrough in technology through its advancements in cognitive assessments. It has contributed significantly in improving diagnostic of brain health which was sufficiently challenged in the past. DCTClock, a proprietary assessment tool of Linus health in brain imaging, has incorporated the use of 50 metrics with AI and advances in neuroscience to reimagine the core of diagnostics in cognitive tests of human brain (Linus Health, 2023). Contrarily, PathAI was a diagnostic tool designed to assist pathologist for early detection of cancer and readily marginalize practitioner's error pertinent to cancer detection. PathAI has created a network of 450 pathologists with a data leverage of 150 million annotations that are aimed to improve pathologists experience in examining patient tissue samples. With sufficient advancement in technology, both Linus health and PathAI has transformed medical practice through incorporation of AI.

Diagnostic of dementia is a complicated procedure which limits practitioner's ability to treat it in initial stage to assist in controlling its spread over the brain. Through Digital Clock and Recall (DCR) of Linus health, practitioners are able to detect symptoms of dementia (Linus Health, 2023). Linus health is also responsible of meeting cognitive care need among adults while focusing on marginalizing the time taken for tests which vacant time space for critical clinical activities. DCR also detects signs of impairment through AI in an optimized time limit of 3 minutes which sufficiently assists practitioners in resorting to AI for better testing results. Through AI, the entire process is automated and require minimal human interference for test results. Therefore, Linus health has gathered the desired success in the US for cognitive assessments. Based on the analysis made by DCR, Linus health provides a dashboard with recommendations to improve patient's health. Each of its recommendation is powered by efficient use of AI training and ML to empower accuracy and effectiveness of its recommendation. Therefore, it is perceived to be among the important developments of AI for practitioners in bridging the quality gap.

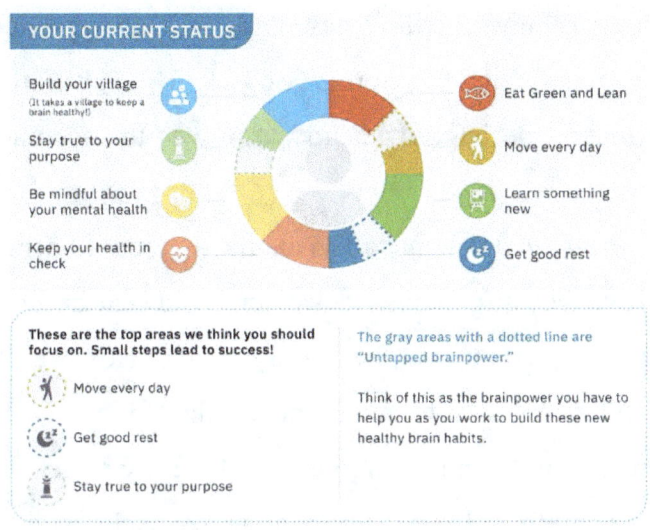

Figure 8 Screenshot of Dashboard (Linus Health, 2023)

Life and death in patient care are determined by gap between practitioner and patient along with the time taken for a practitioner to treat or operate a patient. However, managerial gaps often presented biased views on understanding of urgency for distinct patients increasing the gap between two stakeholders. Viz.ai provided a unique managerial solution for patient management which was aimed to marginalize and control the gap between practitioners and patients depending on the level of urgency detected through AI. Viz.ai incorporates the use of FDA-cleared algorithms for efficient interpretation of CT scans, electrocardiogram (EKGs), and echocardiograms while providing real time insights and diagnostic assessment for efficient patient care (Viz.ai, 2023). Viz.ai specializes in radiology, neuro, cardio, vascular, and trauma. It has readily redefined the norms of AI in healthcare for practitioners and has sufficiently improved the accuracy of diagnostics.

Among the long lasted battle of practitioners was against cancer in patients. It was analyzed that cancer and tumor in early stages can be readily treated. However, their early detection was found to be hurdled due to lack of patient care and complication caused by early stage cancer.

Therefore, Freenome empowered healthcare sector with a blood test routine which checks for biomarkers of tumor and non-tumor based sources. The AI-based technology assists practitioners in early diagnostic of cancer and its elimination from the source through corrective surgery and treatment measures which may include the use of biopsy, chemotherapy and cancer removal surgeries. However, each of the preceding surgical measures complicate themselves with growing stage of cancer. Thus, through the use of Freenome, the inclusion of early stage detection readily trivializes surgical measures to treat cancer.

The criticality and contribution of redundant tasks such as incorporation of forms during admission and discharge has consumed practitioners (Malhotra et al., 2007). The following figure showed the workflow of redundant tasks incorporated by health practitioners which marginalizes their attention towards their actual job. Thus, healthcare management applications through the usage of AI have developed efficient frameworks to incorporate admission and discharge reports automatically while synchronizing the procedure with EHR for record of patient health history.

Furthermore, it significantly saves time for health practitioners in fulfilling tasks which have no active contribution towards patient's quality satisfaction. Since AI in healthcare is relatively an innovation, it was determined that introduction of AI with such tasks can prove to be an initial step for fulfilment of AI in healthcare. The redundancy in such tasks also takes significant toll on job satisfaction of employees as they are not contributing directly to the cause of quality in healthcare. However, their documentation practices had led to increased knowledge management for extensive patient care.

In contrast, it was determined that integration of AI can automate the process entirely which marginalizes human attention towards redundant tasks.

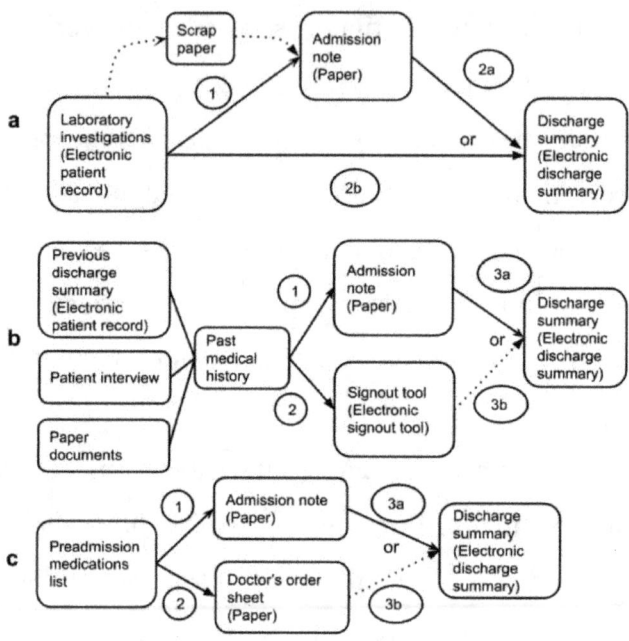

Figure 9 Details of Redundant Task in Healthcare (MacMillan et al., 2016)

The administrative efficiency provided by AI in healthcare sector has corresponded to marginalized errors in documentation process along with scheduling, billing, and patient access to consultants. The non-clinical contribution of AI included automation of administrative tasks, amplifying insight generation, along with fraud, waste and abuse (FWA) detection and prevention (Liu et al., 2016). The size of US healthcare market has benefitted the incorporation of FWA due to inability of healthcare practitioners to detect fraudulent activities on their own. Therefore, there was an increased requirement of addressing FWA through AI and data sciences. Incorporation of data sciences enables an institution to maintain due diligence of supply and demand of health equipment while ensuring that the requirements of patients are adequately met. Amidst Covid-19, due to FWA, several patients were neglected primarily because of inadequate resources within a hospital. Since technology is not entirely embraced by US healthcare sector, a cemented percentage of FWA is yet to be found which could extensively bridge the quality gap in healthcare. Following table shows the action US healthcare sector can take to marginalize FWA through incorporation of AI:

Table 3 Action to take for marginalization of FWA

Actions to take for marginalization of FWA	
Preemptive detection capabilities for FWA detection	Identification of existing paradigms of FWA and their impact on organizational capabilities. It will yield significant advantages to devise an AI interface which detects FWA probability and likelihood beforehand through advanced data

	analytics
Root cause and cost assessment	The root cause and cost assessment strategies enable an organization to practice extensive need realization. Furthermore, empowerment of FWA detection program to detect any new methods of perpetrators of healthcare can lead to significant improvement in due diligence of key resources
Continuous improvements	Feed FWA AI with relevant data on resources and tracking of resources to adequately plan demand in accordance to the need of institution (Rayan, 2019). It will entirely block the presence of FWA in a healthcare setting while bridging quality gap

Marginalization of FWA enables quality incentive practitioners to have extensive ability of resources for better treatment of the patients (Sun et al., 2020). Practitioners in US healthcare were often faced with capacity issues along with resource issues related to patient care due to FWA. However, through incorporation of AI, practitioners will be able to address patient requirement which enhances the perceived quality of healthcare. Contrarily, the existing paradigm dictates that healthcare sector is reliant on good practices of practitioners to bridge quality gap in US healthcare. Through correction facilities of FWA by AI, the availability of resources along with management crisis within US healthcare will significantly reduce (Hayes, 2022). Contrarily, it was argued that the incorporation of AI in non-clinical task is a stepping stone for AI's inclusion in health framework. Since the need realization among practitioners for AI is significantly challenged; therefore, ability of AI can be demonstrated by implementation in non-clinical tasks which can generate desired level of attention of internal stakeholders to marginalize quality gap.

Continuous learning and improvement programs of AI that has been extensively used in the business environment can be readily used to aid practitioners as well. The value of experience among practitioners is graded highly in healthcare; and same is the case with AI (Pianykh et al., 2020). It was determined that AI requires experience to make efficient prediction or solutions for improvement of quality.

However, the realm of experience significantly differs for AI compared to human experience. The human experience requires time and variation of cases; however, in case of AI, it only requires data for better accuracy. Furthermore, human interaction with patients carry a range of dynamic factors that incorporates biasness; however, in case of AI it detaches biasness from decision making.

Therefore, continuous learning programs of AI are perceived to create greater benefits for the health industry. Furthermore, the automated medical image interpretation has also marginalized the range of errors which was presumably found to be 36% in the following figure. However, a significant portion of healthcare practitioners with 28% are yet to believe in the capabilities of AI for bridging quality gap.

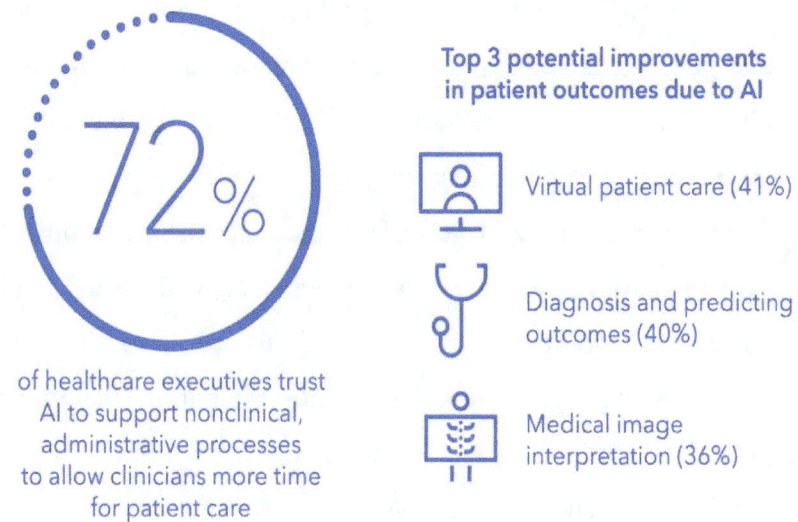

Figure 10 AI's contribution in Healthcare Industry (Medtronic, 2020)

In accordance to the figure above, 72% of the practitioners were benefitted with virtual patient care, diagnosis and predicting outcomes, and medical image interpretation. However, the advantages of AI in clinical arrangements are extensive and also includes symptom analysis, detection of urgency for a patient, research and development (Reddy et al., 2020). Research and development was found to be the key inclusion of AI in healthcare for practitioners amidst mutation of disease causing viruses and bacteria.

AI has exhibited commendable capabilities in researching changes in DNA structure of disease causing viruses which were an extensive limitation for adequate treatment of patient. A disease which may portray similar symptoms as a regular disease may have mutated structure which could not be addressed through conventional medicines, treatment or surgeries.

However, with efficient studies on mutation of viruses through AI, the practitioners can efficiently treat patient according to the level of disease and possible repercussions associated with complication. Covid-19 provided efficient example on mutation of virus complicated enough increase death rate of the country. Thus, it was interpreted that such pandemics can be avoided through advanced researching capabilities offered by AI if it is empowered with desired data set.

Genomic analysis was found to be an extensive disruption of AI and technology in healthcare as it enabled the healthcare to be empowered with genetic coding of DNA for extensive research on disease development within different genetic families (Dias and Tokamani, 2019). It enables the EHR to be extensively empowered in making suggestion to practitioner regarding possible genetic disorder among the patient that could limit the treatment prescribed by doctors.

Furthermore, genomic analysis has significantly empowered early detection of diseases in which the results are used to predetermine possible diseases among the patients through relevant data and predictive analysis (Krause et al., 2021). The practitioners are able to extend their mechanism of treatment and define possible intervention for patient to marginalize materialisation of risk in facing diseases. Furthermore, genomic analysis empowered the healthcare scientists to improve the overall quality of healthcare research.

Conventionally, practitioners were responsible to statistically analyse the data themselves for research settings in healthcare with varying statistical and data analysis expertise. The inclination of healthcare research towards quantitative finding was necessary to cement the results along with probability of success. However, researchers and practitioners were confined with limited abilities to bifurcate anomalies along with limitation in statistical understanding and implementation (Mbonane et al., 2020).

In case of AI, it was noticed that the rigorous data analysis and scientific approach undertaken by technology readily marginalises errors and increases the effectiveness of research. Furthermore, it was noticed that practitioners trusted statistical analysis of AI more than conventional human resources by understanding the limitation and scope of AI in analysis. It enabled practitioners to actively implement research in their daily practice to improve quality of healthcare. With cemented belief in research findings, the learning abilities of practitioners also enhanced along with their ability to practice new methods of patient treatment.

The following table shows a detailed feature of contribution of AI in healthcare which can readily enhance performance of healthcare in the country:

Table 4 Contribution of AI in Healthcare

Informed patient care	Informed patient care can be improved through extensively available data. Conventionally, practitioners were manually viewing EHR for patient's history with healthcare. However, AI develops a swift opinion regarding patient's condition through accessibility of EHR which promotes informed patient care among physicians (Kavitha and Murthy, 2019).
Error reduction	Error detection will be conducted by AI through counterchecking decision of practitioners and providing them

	second opinions regarding their judgement of patient's condition. Figure 1 primarily show cased the inclination of medical errors that were diversified yet easily addressed by AI technologies.
Reducing cost of care	The improvement in appointment scheduling can create a balance between demand and supply of healthcare. As a result, the responsibilities of workforce can be marginalised which can actively contribute to enhanced attention towards highly critical cases in healthcare sector (Matheny et al., 2020).
Doctor-patient engagement	Patients are prone to be more critical of their conditions after their visit to the physicians primarily due to their ability to research and judge a prescription online regarding the troubles they are facing. Therefore, AI can step in as a query addressor for patient inquiries related to their visit

	by highlighting their level of urgency or anxiety to relevant healthcare centres.
Providing contextual relevance	The use of NLP and deep learning can readily relate new medications with old medication prescribed by practitioner to readily determine the improvement or deterioration of health of patients while updating their medical records (Wen et al., 2019).

The drug discovery program powered by AI mutates the molecular structure of advanced medications (Zhou et al., 2022). The need for drug discovery program was defined by the increasing mutation of bacterial diseases along with toxin imbalance in human body (Chen et al., 2020). However, the drug discovery program and development through AI researches extensively on the molecular structure of complex bacteria and uses existing studies to trivialise drug discovery process.

The trivialisation process powered by AI has significantly improved practitioner's effectiveness ratio to treat their respective patients. As a result, the practitioners are extensively firm in their approach to treat patient and the psychological supremacy of the practitioners significantly increases the patient belief in healthcare as well (Chen et al., 2020). Furthermore, drug discovery programs have significantly rectified strategies to study mutation of bacteria through AI as they marginalise the requirement of human intervention in studying and notifying each mutation separately and developing distinctive drug for each mutation.

AI in healthcare has the potential to enhance quality of medical practice by early detection, improve treatment outcomes, increase patient engagement, and make healthcare delivery efficient and accessible. However, it is important to address ethical concerns, data privacy issues, and ensure that AI technologies are integrated in a way that complements the expertise of healthcare professionals while prioritizing patients concern. The pressing issue of patients and practitioners alike is the increasing demands of healthcare in the country (Cyr et al., 2019). It has contributed to deterioration of healthcare mechanism, quality and patient expectation along with motivation of practitioners.

Due to increased work pressure and redundancy on the job, practitioners have shown their disregard with the profession. However, the inclusion of AI has significantly disrupted the healthcare system with significant control over redundant processes while contributing in highly complex procedures such as neuro surgeries and treatment guidelines for complex diseases. Furthermore, its ability to extend research on mutation of diseases and their advancement has also increased the belief of practitioners in healthcare.

Chapter 4:

Contribution of AI in Healthcare for Patients

Practitioners were often found to be confused with multiple symptoms in a patient which led them towards an increased risk of malpractice in diagnostic. However, margin of error significantly increased as per patient's complication and knowledge of practitioner.

Through Buoy Health, making sense of symptoms through AI trained model efficiently provides opinion to practitioners regarding the disease. It also categorizes the complication on levels of self-care and urgent care. It has readily improved the life of patients in addressing the urgency level from their own personal space while marginalizing the burden on US healthcare sector. The inclination of patients towards self-diagnostics were powered through blogs on internet which were only accurate for their particular cases (Al Hakim et al., 2020).

However, with Buoy Health, patients were able to detect the accurate disease they were combating while determining the level of urgency to see a health practitioner.

HealthXL was depicted to be among the core innovations in digital healthcare which has incentivized patients' expectation of quality healthcare. It primarily focused on providing quality feedback to health experts and patients regarding management of patient's illnesses and proven method of treatment. The company extensively believes in building a better digital health framework for efficient patient solution. Furthermore, it emphasizes on choosing a success metric that readily corresponds to realistically interpret the quality gaps in healthcare management (HealthXL, 2023).

The need for digital healthcare is extensively required due to an increased demand of healthcare. Furthermore, the increasing quality gap required digital disruptions which could extensively empower patient knowledge and solutions. Amidst increasing waiting time for public healthcare, digital health solutions can readily pave way to control quality gap by meeting patient's expectations online. The following figure shows some of salient features of HealthXL in providing patient care through technology while connecting practitioners with patient through a professional channel:

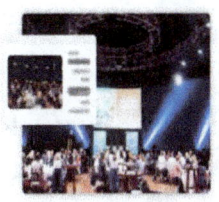 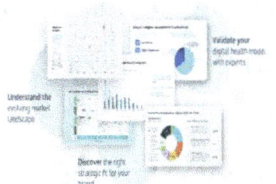 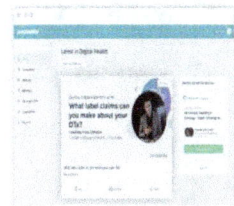

Discuss with leading minds in digital health

Work with dedicated digital health experts

Stay up-to-date with HealthXL's digital health platform.

Figure 11 HealthXL Features (HealthXL, 2023)

Predictive medicine, patient data management and diagnostics, clinical decision making and health service management are among the key aspect of AI which has improved healthcare for patients (Secinaro et al., 2021).

Over 250,000 individuals die annually as a result of medical malpractice primarily comprising of misdiagnosis which is against the good practices of health care (Cha, 2021).

However, through the inclusion of AI in healthcare management, patients are able to efficiently believe in the treatment system powered by technology which does not present any biases against their condition and only provides solution based on their respective condition. Furthermore, in the US, it was determined that racial discrimination in healthcare is an important issue to address as the mortality rate among women belonging to black minority is observed to be 243%, particularly during pregnancy or delivery (ProPublica, 2020).

Thus, inclusion of AI in healthcare can readily enhance patient care as it does incorporate health racial discrimination while providing recommendation. Furthermore, its documented recommendation can assist lawsuits in enhancing the overall capacity of law enforcement to ensure that accusation of malpractice can be efficiently investigated. Thus, AI contributed towards enhanced accountability in healthcare which can significantly enhance the quality of healthcare received in the US.

In the US, the third most common cause of death was found to be medical errors as demonstrated in the figure below. However, usage of technology can significantly mitigate medical errors by providing efficient second opinion to practitioners (Secinaro et al., 2021). Furthermore, the inclusion of knowledge management has sufficiently enhanced quality of healthcare as practitioners are able to incorporate better decision making based on the visualization presented by AI.

It was determined that the dashboards created using AI tools including Linus Health among many others significantly enhances patient's beliefs in practitioner's recommendation and rejuvenates their trust in US healthcare. Contrarily, as per the figure below, 13% depreciation in death rates can be achieved through bridging quality gaps within US healthcare (Cha, 2021).

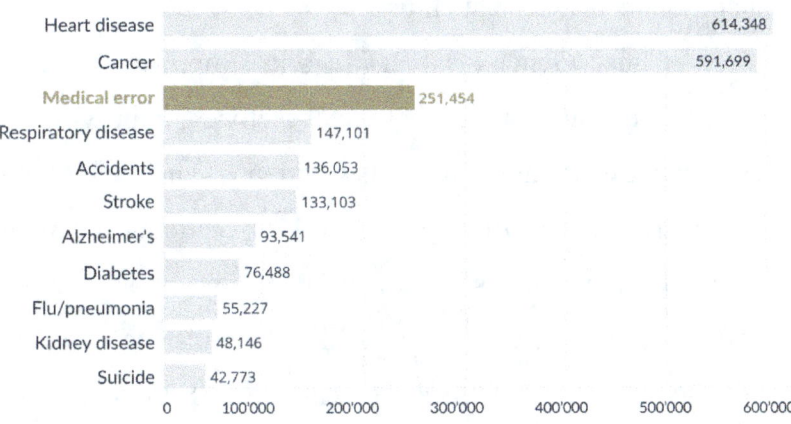

Figure 12 Cause of Death in US (Cha, 2021)

Genetika+, a company established in 2018 operating from Tel Aviv, Israel; is known to have breakthrough research in prescription of anti-depressants through AI which can comprehensively redefine the usage antidepressants and possible misuse (Lisbona, 2023). The company currently researches stem cells and create an environment of brain cells to observe antidepressant reaction on the environment.

As a result, the company will be able to tailor antidepressant drugs for patients rightly according to their needs to marginalize side-effects along with increasing the durability and popularity of antidepressant drugs. Currently, the patients are exposed to negativities associated with antidepressant drugs which leads them to incorporate as their last choice.

Thus, Genetika+ can readily empower patient's health care quality in psychological sector by improving the effectiveness of antidepressants through AI and technology. The alarming rate of increase of 1798 patients' death in 2000 to 5859 patients' death in 2021 from antidepressant over dosage required initiatives like Genetika+ to empower healthcare sector in controlling death rates (Elflein, 2023).

Remote healthcare offered by aforementioned companies have increased convenience for the patients. There was an increased burden on patient transportation through ambulances primarily due to false alarms among the patient which could have been marginalized with remote healthcare. However, conventional online health platforms readily recommended presence of a doctor's opinion prior to any decision due to which patients rushed to the hospitals in urgency while depreciating their perceived quality of healthcare.

Through remote healthcare, AI can easily interpret patient symptoms to gain an insight on their level of urgency and requirement of hospital visits. Synchronization with nearest hospital facility can also enable the hospital to prepare for the patient beforehand to give them timely treatment. It was noticed that the controlled time spent within hospital facility yielded greater perception of quality among the patients (Umoke et al., 2020).

Therefore, remote healthcare can significantly marginalize quality gaps between perception of the patients and quality of healthcare delivered by practitioners. Furthermore, through remote consultation through AI, patients can control their periodic visits to consultants as it is among the controlling factors of healthcare quality since it occupies time of consultants in periodic visits.

Sufficient training of AI through machine learning (ML) and deep learning (DL) enables AI to analyze test reports incorporated from patient history through ultrasound, MRI, and numerous other tests to predetermine diseases among a patient or remain informed about the possibility of a disease which may assist practitioner in taking preemptive measures (Ahsan et al., 2022).

ML and DL algorithms also interpret neural networks extensively while evaluating sensory measures of each node of neural network to develop an understanding of complication in a patient. It was noticed that support vector machine (SVM) in ML and convolutional neural network (CNN) in DL are extensively used techniques for early diagnosis of neural complications (Han et al., 2021).

Despite the complication of procedure, AI is trained to incorporate data from EHR to maintain the interest of practitioners in taking preemptive measures. Furthermore, such practices of cautious method have enabled patients to revitalize their trust in medical institutions. However, the SVM, ML and CNN in DL are costly to implement while a significant portion of practitioners have opposed automated diagnostic likelihood method which has raised a challenge for quality improvement in US healthcare. It was argued that automated checks of diagnostics can also increase rate of false alarms which may increase the burden on US healthcare.

The astounding ratio of google search regarding health constitute of 5% of its total search queries by users (Patel, 2023). However, the number of website, articles and blogs portrayed on google were only found to be accurate for case specific results. Google search results analyses the choices of keyword of users to portray results from worldwide web.

Contrarily, the case of enquirer may be different than the case portrayed on the web which may create a needless sense of urgency among the patient (Patel, 2023). Furthermore, the search results of accredited healthcare platforms always motivate patients to consult with their physicians on urgency. Therefore, a need for AI chatbot was required which efficiently engaged with customers and provided instant response to general queries (Athota et al., 2020). Furthermore, AI chatbot can align appointments and scheduling of patient to the nearest healthcare facility based on their urgency through a centralized platform. The following figure demonstrates possible properties of AI chatbot which can be trivially implemented in American healthcare sector:

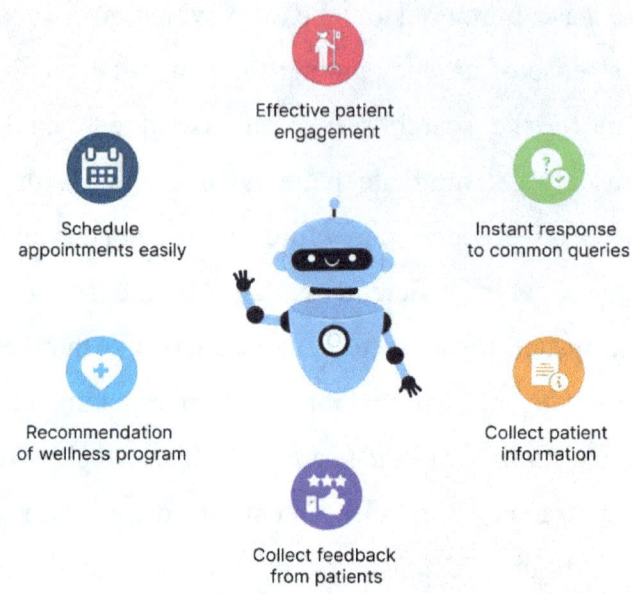

Practitioners rating of patient care rated by their respective patient was found to be linked with availability of physicians. An average wait time for 5-star rating doctors was found to be 13 minutes and 17 seconds while 1-star rating doctors had a waiting time of over 34 minutes and 11 seconds in accordance to the table below (Mattio, 2018).

Therefore, waiting time was found to be critical in terms of healthcare rating (Mattio, 2018). In New York, 30% of the patients walked out of an appointment due to long waits which is critical for healthcare rating and challenges the entire concept of healthcare accessibility. Thus, there was an increasing need to re-establish control of patient appointments via use of chatbots. Contrarily, the presence of chatbots and increased efficiency of the practitioners in healthcare lowered the wait time for patients by 22 seconds (Mattio, 2018). As a result, it was proven that widespread integration of AI chatbots through centralised stream of healthcare can exponentially reduce wait time which is critical for sustainability for healthcare and improves patient lives in terms of accessibility.

Wait Time Effect on Doctor Rating

Star Rating	Average Wait Time
5	13 min, 17 sec
4	21 min, 32 sec
3	22 min, 11 sec
2	29 min, 34 sec
1	34 min, 11 sec

Figure 14 Average Waiting Time for Patients in Relation to Physician's Rating (Mattio, 2018)

The inclination of wait time in healthcare across states differed significantly due to burdened healthcare facilities with increased demand. Wisconsin and New Hampshire were among the key states to be negatively responding to the increasing need of healthcare urgency (Hubers et al., 2020).

Their inability to adapt to technological reforms was investigated to be among the common reason for increased wait time. Furthermore, the speculation and pressure associated with increased demand of healthcare further contributed to stress level for practitioners. As a result, the recovery of patient was readily reduced which created an imbalance in the increasing demand for healthcare.

In accordance to the policy makers, the cities enlisted in the figure below were prioritised for attention for incorporation of AI and technology to improve appointment structure while monitoring the urgency level for patients (Mattio, 2018). The new policy framework allowed practitioners to bypass conventional scheduling system to treat patients with higher level of urgency (Napi et al., 2019). However, the new approach created a significant gap due to subjective approach of practitioners which readily challenged the qualitative approach undertaken by practitioners.

2018 Cities with Shortest Wait Time

City	Average Wait Time
Milwaukee	14 min, 35 sec
Seattle	14 min, 38 sec
Saint Paul	14 min, 43 sec
Minneapolis	14 min, 55 sec
Portland	15 min, 6 sec

2018 Cities with Longest Wait Time

City	Average Wait Time
El Paso	26 min, 50 sec
Memphis	23 min, 44 sec
Miami	22 min, 29 sec
Las Vegas	21 min, 19 sec
Fort Worth	21 min, 1 sec

Figure 15 Longest and Shortest Wait Time in accordance to Cities (Mattio, 2018)

Pharmaceutical companies were heavily reliant on face-to-face meeting between practitioners and patients for their business revenue. However, the presence of pandemic and imposition of lockdown due to Covid-19 enabled the need for a digital disruption in healthcare industry.

Therefore, an Omni channel engagement in pharmaceutical companies was followed which provided an inclusive digital experience for patient treatment (Proskurnina et al., 2021).

The figure below shows the benefits associated with Omni channel engagement and determined that the personalised patient experience increases their accessibility towards healthcare and abundant demand of healthcare in the region is efficiently met by an automated supply of AI practitioners (Shaheen, 2021). Furthermore, it was noticed that their ability to deal with redundant tasks allowed practitioner to spend more time on effective research and development which enhances the belief in healthcare for patients.

The difference in traditional online queries and Omni channel system is the ability to provide personalised experience for patients which enhances their belief in healthcare mechanism across the US (Kavitha and Murthy, 2019).

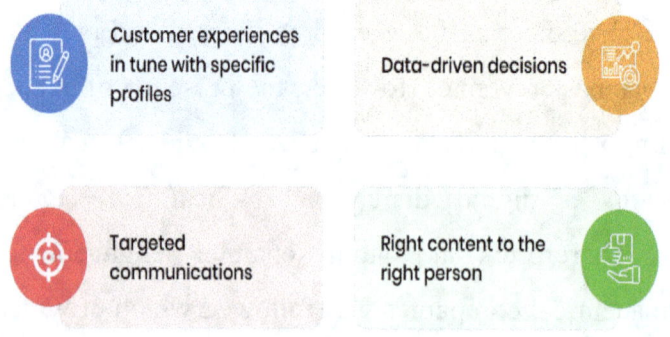

Figure 16 Benefits of Omni channel engagement in Pharma (Singh, 2023)

Key elements of Omni channel marketing strategy by pharmaceuticals include the following points:

- **Focus on virtual care of medicine:** The new modes of engagement featuring chat bots powered by NLP has readily increased prospects of healthcare within the region.

- **Optimisation across channels:** The optimisation of Omni channels can sufficiently improve healthcare by improving accessibility across all channels of healthcare (Proskurnina et al., 2021).

- **Personalisation:** The personalised aspect of AI technologies via chatbot can enhance the level of trust placed by patients on healthcare system across the country (Kavitha and Murthy, 2019).

- **Performance measurement:** Performance measurement through a centralised channel can provide an efficient report on all constituencies of healthcare.

- **Data-driven decisions**: Usage of digital disruption in healthcare can centralise data collection strategies which can improve and improvise data driven decision making (Proskurnina et al., 2021).

Patient data management, public health insights and predictive analytics have been observed as a key to improve patient's belief in healthcare (Dimitrov, 2019). The automated assistance in data management through EHR has provided significant enhancement on the quality of communication between doctors and patients. Patients were found to press more on their existing complications which may deter practitioner's interest from the underlying problem in patient's health. However, through increased access to health records and key insights from AI, practitioners can readily expand their focus on patient's complication (Yaqoob et al., 2021).

Furthermore, the public health insights enable the patient to look for any complication beforehand in their body which enhances their belief in healthcare system. Amidst Covid-19, patients were restricted to visit their respective health facilities unless direly needed. However, public health insights enabled the practitioners to increase their accessibility towards the patients while enhancing their experience towards US healthcare. As a result, patient data management and public health insights have resulted in enhanced quality experience of US healthcare.

The following figure shows the process of predictive analytics incorporated by healthcare sector.

Predictive analytics primarily inclines itself on the definition, aim and objective of the project (Van Calster et al., 2019).

Furthermore, it emphasizes on data collection, screening, building and testing a model prior to establishment of results that could be used improve quality of US healthcare by early detection of advanced diseases.

The inclination of predictive analytics in US healthcare contributes to increased research and development. Conventionally, research and development in healthcare was extensively focused on incorporating samples for studies which often increased the cost of experimentation in the field of medicine (Galetski and Katsaliaki, 2020).

However, through evident data and incorporating the use of AI in data management, the research and development sector has marginalized its cost of research (Van Calster et al., 2019). Therefore, increased findings in literature and research has enabled the healthcare practitioner to be critical of patient's health in modernized system. Furthermore, through the usage of predictive analytics, practitioners have reduced the wait time for patients as they establish a pre-conceived judgement on patient health using the result of predictive analytics while checking for its correctness.

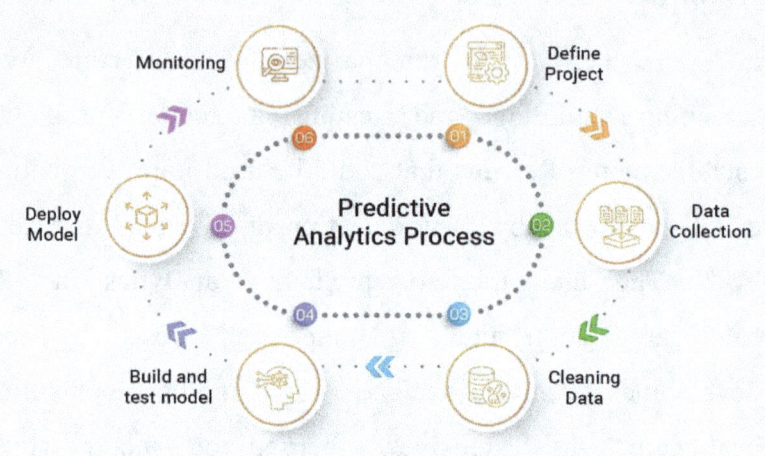

Figure 17 Predictive Analytics Process (Van Calster et al., 2019)

The tailored intervention through predictive analytics process has readily enhanced patient's belief in healthcare regarding the quality of insights provided by respective practitioners (Purba et al., 2019). The inclination of patients towards tested treatment in healthcare statistically yields more satisfaction compared to new treatment.

Furthermore, it was analyzed that the predictive analysis procedure rigorously tests and monitor new model of health treatment prior to practice which enhances the belief of practitioners and patients alike. The patients were increasingly reliant on technology of procedures and AI further developed its stance in tailoring patient treatment plan through accessing their medical history. Conventional medical paradigm rested highly within the medication side-effects which were often neglected by practitioners which led to complications.

However, through AI, the assessment of patient medication in accordance to their medical history has increased the effectiveness of treatment on the patient and enhanced overall quality of healthcare (Babel et al., 2021). Thus, AI has played a significant role in bridging gap of healthcare in the US by increasing patients' belief in technology and healthcare through statistical and consultative intervention.

A modernised approach towards predictive analytics in healthcare involves 4 stages that includes describe, diagnose, predict and prescribe (Purba et al., 2019). The stage of prediction and prescription are determined to be the crucial stages which are considered to be dynamic due to range of practitioners' experience associated with a particular disease. A practitioner may approach a disease differently based on their prior experience of drug reaction among the patients enabling to mitigate the risks associated with treatment or prescription errors.

However, in case of newly exposed practitioner, their treatment would involve risk and possible intrusion of drug side effects that may challenge quality of healthcare. Thus, the usage of technology to standardize experiential progress among the practitioners is imminent that improves quality of healthcare and marginalize the utilization of key resources in determining possible treatment and methods.

Chapter 5:

Conclusion

Increase in quality gap in healthcare was found to be associated with following factors which included errors related to treatment, obstetrics, medication, surgery, anesthesia, and diagnostics. Each of the preceding errors were found to be marginalized through technological innovations and embracement in the healthcare sector.

Introduction and empowerment of AI in healthcare management can alleviate the change management resistance among the practitioners regarding usage of technology in healthcare. Primarily, the practitioners were found to have invested themselves in getting industry related expertise to increase their employability which reduced their focus towards technological innovations.

However, the persistence of fields such as bio-medical engineering enabled healthcare sector to realize the importance of technology in bridging quality gaps. The unprecedented benefits of AI inclusion in healthcare contribute to enhanced patient care, marginalized medical errors through incorporation of EHR, patient education, and reduction in cost of healthcare. The enhanced ability of industry to improvise their healthcare delivery process through technology can enhance their efficiency of quality in healthcare.

The unreported errors by the patient corresponded to the primary defense of practitioners against claims of malpractice or undermined healthcare quality. However, through EHR and incorporation of machine learning, patient's history can be accessed that can contribute to the practitioner's ability to find a suitable treatment. Furthermore, it enhances practitioners' trust in technological expertise in their industry which can pave way for further development in automation of treatment processes and recommendation that can improve ability of the industry to address increasing healthcare demands. The wait time in diversified region of the US was found to be among the common reason for low rated healthcare.

Therefore, technological incorporation and better resource management can enable the practitioners to focus their expertise on urgent patient care. Companies like Genetika+ have made breakthrough research to marginalize misdiagnosis by practitioners while prescribing drugs. Deep learning, machine learning in collaboration with AI has instigated significant advancements in the field of research of medicine.

The alarming appraisal of quality gaps in healthcare have been redirected towards technology for immediate solutions. The inclination of US government to incorporate AI in healthcare management has addressed the diversified demands of quality enhancement procedures including general wait time for patients, virtual assistance of patients from home, and significant advancements to enhance practitioner's capabilities associated with patients' care.

However, the increasing demand of technology is met with the limited expertise of practitioners to incorporate technologies in their daily lives. Thus, AI was noticed as an advancement which could enable practitioners to embrace usage of technology with a convenient user interface as observed in figures chapter 2 and 3. It enables practitioners to focus on patient's progress associated with their disease while incorporating key insights from AI advancement tools such as HealthXL, PathAi and several others. As a result, practitioners are able to make swift judgement regarding patients' condition allowing them to close the quality gap within healthcare.

Historically, it has been assumed that the healthcare sector can never meet expectation of the patients due to inevitable death. However, quality gaps in healthcare are evident which can be filled by technology to achieve higher quality.

AI, ML and data management of EHR has significantly advanced patient management activities from scheduling appointments to scanning history of patient complication to meet their expectations. However, the cost of AI and ML for hospital management in the US is significantly high due to increasing demand of services.

Furthermore, technological innovations are not controlled or liberated within the healthcare industry but is offered as a product from technological services industry. As a result, the cost of technological enhancement in healthcare is significantly higher. Contrarily, majority of healthcare facilities in the US are publicly operated. Thus, the budget for technological innovation, in terms of opportunity cost, was found to be affordable. However, experimentation and maturity of new healthcare models is found challenging due to lack of practitioner expertise in the product.

Technological innovations in the healthcare industry such as diagnostic tools have readily empowered practitioners in taking decisive actions against patient's complication.

Traditionally, practitioners were constraint with possible repercussion of their treatment which hindered their approach. However, with efficient collaboration and diagnostics from health records of patients, AI can readily empower practitioner approach to control treatment mechanism and marginalize malpractice claims to empower quality. 5.1% of medical malpractice due to prescription, 2.5% anesthesia related errors and 24.1% surgery related errors can be significantly mitigated through AI and its incorporation in healthcare industry that can excessively bridge the quality gaps.

However, the opportunity cost associated with AI implementation along with resistance to change management has readily resisted the growth of technology in healthcare. Thus, government's intervention is required through HIPPA and PPACA which can enhance the accountability of technological innovation at healthcare centers. Since the proven improvement of quality through AI and patient management, the success of enhanced technological innovation in healthcare is imminent.

The facilitation of technology has assisted in efficient patient management in accordance to their level of urgencies. Patient feedback on healthcare was found to deteriorate after their increased waiting time and compromised health at the time of treatment or consultation which resulted in significant quality gaps. Preliminary technological inclusion in pre-assistive consultation through AI has readily enabled the patients to trust in US healthcare sector which has increased its perceived quality in the recent past.

However, the cases regarding malpractice and traditional norms in the industry are still a challenge which has to be readily addressed. Technology is the comprehensive answer to healthcare quality questions. Thus, incorporation of AI does not only benefit patients but also assist practitioners in incorporating a decisive approach to treat their respective patients.

The positive and formidable relationship shared between technology and healthcare is strengthened due to technology's assistance in reducing practitioner related error and providing a rechecking measure. It enables the practitioner to countercheck their decision based on the available information. However, the preliminary condition of improvement is the ability of practitioner to accept technology and change management. Otherwise, the technological influence will only marginalize practitioner performance. As a result, in the US, technological skills are optimally focused in coursework of aspiring medical practitioners.

Furthermore, a more inclusive environment in healthcare industry is created where technical expertise of biomedical engineers, physicians and researchers collaborate among each other to equip the industry with breakthrough innovations. The existing innovations including PathAI and Genetika+ are a result of technological advancement with controlled involvement of practitioners in the initial stages of project. However, if the project were to involve doctors and practitioner in their research and development of the application, the process of completing the application with effectiveness may have been catalyzed.

Compliance of quality standards in healthcare were often marginalized due to extensive history of the patients along with practitioner's urgency to make a decision based on patient's sensitivity. However, through technology and better accessibility of EHR through centralized channel enabled the practitioner to take a glance at the patient history and used AI to analyze their prior health record to recommend new tests based on the available data with AI.

Thus, technology primarily enables practitioners with a direction to investigate patient's health and re-strategize their treatment plans. AR has also empowered the trends in surgery with effective training methodologies to train new surgeons regarding possible procedures and repercussion prior to surgery. Since surgery related errors caused 24.1% of malpractice claims in the US that proved to be fatal for patients; AR empowers practitioners to find possible errors in their practice and mitigation strategies to increase their respective effectiveness.

In pursuit of technological innovation focused through AI, healthcare industry has readily diversified their focus from the possible advantages offered by AR in the field of surgery and research. It is recommended that the AR functionalities are used extensively in healthcare apart from training their new surgeons and assist their research based on virtual reality (VR) as well. It will enable practitioners to reduce their errors in surgery while benefitting the mortality rate in operation room. The majority of fatal errors in patient recovery processes generate from operation room. Therefore, usage of AR can significantly marginalize the errors associated with surgeon while allowing them to enhance their precision without experimenting on a human body.

Furthermore, AR in collaboration with biomedical engineers can readily automate the surgery aspect within the industry as well.

The evolution of health information technology (HIT) in the recent past has been a breakthrough innovation for decision making and support mechanism to bridge quality gaps in healthcare. Contrarily, the research and development in the field of technology and healthcare is significantly constricted by practitioners' lack of ability to incorporate technology. As a result, the process and evolution of HIT is hindered by existing practices within the industry.

The inclination of PPACA and other health intermediaries of the US have urged institutions to diversify their operational capabilities to accept technological innovation in their respective practices. During the initial stages, the government had urged institutions to automate their appointment mechanism to control waiting time for the patients. Thus, similar methods must be incorporated by the government to urge the hospitals to embrace technological innovations in the healthcare industry.

As a result, the inclusion of AI has been observed as a resource in itself which promises to be an integral part of US healthcare services in future. The resourcefulness of AI in contemplating innovation in medicine and healthcare has empowered the industry to control their dependence on human resources and standardize healthcare across the country.

It is among the rising issues where the practitioners are not able to standardize their attention towards patients, compromising on the overall quality of healthcare. With AI as an active resource in healthcare industry, it is determined that institutions can increasingly control their dependency on human practitioner while the practitioners themselves can incorporate the support of AI for enhanced decision making. It is among the fields that require humanized feedback for better determination of patient health; and the evolution of HIT along with AI has been providing better efficiency in decision making to enhance the quality of healthcare offered in the US. Therefore, we determine AI as a doctor for our future.

References

Ahn, E. J., Kim, H. J., Kim, K. W., Choi, H. R., Kang, H., & Bang, S. R. (2019). Comparison of general anesthesia and regional anesthesia in terms of mortality and complications in elderly patients with hip fracture: a nationwide population-based study. *BMJ open*, *9*(9), e029245.

Ahsan, M. M., Luna, S. A., & Siddique, Z. (2022, March). Machine-learning-based disease diagnosis: A comprehensive review. In *Healthcare* (Vol. 10, No. 3, p. 541). MDPI.

Akhtar, N., Singh, V., Yusuf, M., & Khan, R. A. (2020). Non-invasive drug delivery technology: Development and current status of transdermal drug delivery devices, techniques and biomedical applications. *Biomedical Engineering/Biomedizinische Technik*, *65*(3), 243-272.

Al Hakim, R. R., Rusdi, E., & Setiawan, M. A. (2020). Android based expert system application for diagnose COVID-19 disease: Cases study of banyumas regency. *J Int Comp & He Inf*, *1*(2).

AltexSoft (2021) *Natural language processing in healthcare: Using text analysis for medical documentation and decision-making, AltexSoft.* Available at: https://www.altexsoft.com/blog/nlp-healthcare/ (Accessed: 15 July 2023).

Amann, J., Blasimme, A., Vayena, E., Frey, D., & Madai, V. I. (2020). Explainability for artificial intelligence in healthcare: a multidisciplinary perspective. *BMC medical informatics and decision making, 20*(1), 1-9.

American Medical Association (2023) *Trends in health care spending, American Medical Association.* Available at: https://www.ama-assn.org/about/research/trends-health-care-spending#:~:text=Health%20spending%20in%20the%20U.S.,2020%20(10.3%25%20percent). (Accessed: 11 July 2023).

Athota, L., Shukla, V. K., Pandey, N., & Rana, A. (2020, June). Chatbot for healthcare system using artificial intelligence. In *2020 8th International conference on reliability, infocom technologies and optimization (trends and future directions)(ICRITO)* (pp. 619-622). IEEE.

Awad, A., Trenfield, S. J., Pollard, T. D., Ong, J. J., Elbadawi, M., McCoubrey, L. E., ... & Basit, A. W. (2021). Connected healthcare: Improving patient care using digital health technologies. *Advanced Drug Delivery Reviews*, *178*, 113958.

Babel, A., Taneja, R., Mondello Malvestiti, F., Monaco, A., & Donde, S. (2021). Artificial intelligence solutions to increase medication adherence in patients with non-communicable diseases. *Frontiers in Digital Health*, *3*, 669869.

Benítez, M. A., Velasco, C., Sequeira, A. R., Henríquez, J., Menezes, F. M., & Paolucci, F. (2020). Responses to COVID-19 in five Latin American countries. *Health policy and technology*, *9*(4), 525-559.

Bontemps-Hommen, C. M. M. L., Baart, A., & Vosman, F. T. H. (2019). Practical wisdom in complex medical practices: a critical proposal. *Medicine, Health Care and Philosophy*, *22*, 95-105.

Bookman, K., & Zane, R. D. (2020). Surviving a medical malpractice lawsuit. *Emergency Medicine Clinics*, *38*(2), 539-548.

Burki, T. (2019). GP at hand: a digital revolution for health care provision?. *The Lancet*, *394*(10197), 457-460.

Cha, A.E. (2021) *Researchers: Medical errors now third leading cause of death in United States, The Washington Post.* Available at: https://www.washingtonpost.com/news/to-your-health/wp/2016/05/03/researchers-medical-errors-now-third-leading-cause-of-death-in-united-states/ (Accessed: 15 July 2023).

Chen, B., Garmire, L., Calvisi, D. F., Chua, M. S., Kelley, R. K., & Chen, X. (2020). Harnessing big 'omics' data and AI for drug discovery in hepatocellular carcinoma. *Nature Reviews Gastroenterology & Hepatology, 17*(4), 238-251.

Chen, M., & Decary, M. (2020, January). Artificial intelligence in healthcare: An essential guide for health leaders. In *Healthcare management forum* (Vol. 33, No. 1, pp. 10-18). Sage CA: Los Angeles, CA: SAGE Publications.

Cyr, M. E., Etchin, A. G., Guthrie, B. J., & Benneyan, J. C. (2019). Access to specialty healthcare in urban versus rural US populations: a systematic literature review. *BMC health services research, 19*(1), 1-17.

DeBord, L. C., Patel, V., Braun, T. L., & Dao Jr, H. (2018). Social media in dermatology: clinical relevance, academic value, and trends across platforms. *Journal of Dermatological Treatment.*

Deloitte (2023) *Cloud Solutions for Health Care: Deloitte us, Deloitte United States.* Available at: https://www2.deloitte.com/us/en/pages/consulting/art icles/healthcare-cloud-solutions.html?id=us%3A2ps%3A3gl%3Achep24%3Aawa%3Acons%3A071823%3Ahealthcare+technology%3Ab%3Ac%3Akwd-16027986&gclid=Cj0KCQjw5f2lBhCkARIsAHeTvl gfJttaERlfAv2eQjLrIDukU2udWagRxERPEKJzb-dMA1luSkI0MfIaAnfEEALw_wcB (Accessed: 26 July 2023).

Dias, R., & Torkamani, A. (2019). Artificial intelligence in clinical and genomic diagnostics. *Genome medicine, 11*(1), 1-12.

Dimetman, N. (2022) *35 medical malpractice statistics for 2022, Just Great Lawyers.* Available at: https://www.justgreatlawyers.com/legal-guides/medical-malpractice-statistics (Accessed: 17 July 2023).

Dimitrov, D. V. (2019). Blockchain applications for healthcare data management. *Healthcare informatics research, 25*(1), 51-56.

El Khatib, M., Hamidi, S., Al Ameeri, I., Al Zaabi, H., & Al Marqab, R. (2022). Digital disruption and big data in healthcare-opportunities and challenges. *ClinicoEconomics and Outcomes Research*, 563-574.

Elflein, J. (2023) *Antidepressant overdose deaths U.S. 1999-2021, Statista.* Available at: https://www.statista.com/statistics/895959/antidepressant-overdose-deaths-us/#:~:text=Number%20of%20antidepressant%20overdose%20deaths%20U.S.%201999%2D2021&text=In%202021%2C%20there%20were%20an,U.S.%20from%201999%20to%202021. (Accessed: 22 July 2023).

El-Gazzar, R., & Stendal, K. (2020). Blockchain in health care: hope or hype?. *Journal of Medical Internet Research*, *22*(7), e17199.

ForeSee Medical (2023) *Artificial Intelligence (AI) in Healthcare & Hospitals, ForeSee Medical.* Available at: https://www.foreseemed.com/artificial-intelligence-in-healthcare (Accessed: 15 July 2023).

Galetsi, P., & Katsaliaki, K. (2020). A review of the literature on big data analytics in healthcare. *Journal of the Operational Research Society*, *71*(10), 1511-1529.

Gobel, B. (2022) *Medical malpractice statistics 2022: Ogg, Murphy & Perkosky, Ogg, Murphy & Perkosky, P.C.* Available at: https://yourpghlawyer.com/medical-malpractice-statistics-2022/ (Accessed: 10 July 2023).

Han, T., Zhang, L., Yin, Z., & Tan, A. C. (2021). Rolling bearing fault diagnosis with combined convolutional neural networks and support vector machine. *Measurement*, *177*, 109022.

Hasikin, K., Lai, K. W., Satapathy, S. C., Sabanci, K., & Aslan, M. F. (2023). Emerging applications of text analytics and natural language processing in healthcare. *Frontiers in Digital Health*, *5*, 1227948.

Hayes, S. A. (2022). The Three Most Misunderstood Words in Health Care: Fraud, Waste and Abuse. *Benefits Quarterly*, *38*(4).

HealthXL (2023) *Digital Health Intelligence Platform & Community*, *HealthXL*. Available at: https://www.healthxl.com/ (Accessed: 15 July 2023).

Hubers, J., Sonnenberg, A., Gopal, D., Weiss, J., Holobyn, T., & Soni, A. (2020). Trends in wait time for colorectal cancer screening and diagnosis 2013-2016. *Clinical and Translational Gastroenterology, 11*(1).

Iterative Health (2023) *Creating a brighter future for GI care., Iterative Health.* Available at: https://iterative.health/products/ (Accessed: 26 July 2023).

Kamal, S. A., Shafiq, M., & Kakria, P. (2020). Investigating acceptance of telemedicine services through an extended technology acceptance model (TAM). *Technology in Society, 60*, 101212.

Kavitha, B. R., & Murthy, C. R. (2019). Chatbot for healthcare system using Artificial Intelligence. *Int J Adv Res Ideas Innov Technol, 5*, 1304-1307.

Kompa, B., Snoek, J., & Beam, A. L. (2021). Second opinion needed: communicating uncertainty in medical machine learning. *NPJ Digital Medicine, 4*(1), 4.

Krause, T., Jolkver, E., Bruchhaus, S., Kramer, M., & Hemmje, M. (2021, December). GenDAI–AI-Assisted Laboratory Diagnostics for Genomic Applications. In *2021 IEEE International Conference on Bioinformatics and Biomedicine (BIBM)* (pp. 2253-2258). IEEE.

Lee, D., & Yoon, S. N. (2021). Application of artificial intelligence-based technologies in the healthcare industry: Opportunities and challenges. *International Journal of Environmental Research and Public Health, 18*(1), 271.

Linus Health (2023) *Home, Linus Health.* Available at: https://linushealth.com/ (Accessed: 11 July 2023).

Lisbona, N. (2023) *How artificial intelligence is matching drugs to patients, BBC News.* Available at: https://www.bbc.com/news/business-65260592 (Accessed: 22 July 2023).

Liu, J., Bier, E., Wilson, A., Guerra-Gomez, J. A., Honda, T., Sricharan, K., ... & Davies, D. (2016). Graph analysis for detecting fraud, waste, and abuse in healthcare data. *Ai Magazine, 37*(2), 33-46.

MacMillan, T. E., Slessarev, M., & Etchells, E. (2016). eWasted time: Redundant work during hospital admission and discharge. *Health informatics journal, 22*(1), 60-66.

Malhotra, S., Jordan, D., Shortliffe, E., & Patel, V. L. (2007). Workflow modeling in critical care: piecing together your own puzzle. *Journal of biomedical informatics, 40*(2), 81-92.

Manougian, T., & Zangbar, B. (2022). Analgesia and Anesthesia. *Surgical Critical Care and Emergency Surgery: Clinical Questions and Answers*, 123-135.

Matheny, M. E., Whicher, D., & Israni, S. T. (2020). Artificial intelligence in health care: a report from the National Academy of Medicine. *Jama*, *323*(6), 509-510.

Mattio, R. (2018) *9th Annual vitals wait time report released, Business Wire*. Available at: https://www.businesswire.com/news/home/2018032 2005683/en/9th-Annual-Vitals-Wait-Time-Report-Released (Accessed: 17 August 2023).

Mbonane, T. P., & Naicker, N. (2020). Knowledge, attitude and practices of environmental health practitioners conducting food-borne disease outbreak investigation at a local municipality in Gauteng province, South Africa. *Health SA Gesondheid*, *25*.

McKendrick, M., Yang, S., & McLeod, G. A. (2021). The use of artificial intelligence and robotics in regional anesthesia. *Anaesthesia*, *76*, 171-181.

Medtronic. (2020). *5 Ways Artificial Intelligence is transforming healthcare, Medtronic*. Available at: https://www.medtronic.com/us-en/our-company/ai-healthcare-technology-solutions.html (Accessed: 05 August 2023).

Morley, J., Machado, C. C., Burr, C., Cowls, J., Joshi, I., Taddeo, M., & Floridi, L. (2020). The ethics of AI in health care: a mapping review. *Social Science & Medicine, 260*, 113172.

Murala, D. K., Panda, S. K., & Sahoo, S. K. (2023). Securing electronic health record system in cloud environment using blockchain technology. In *Recent advances in blockchain technology: real-world applications* (pp. 89-116). Cham: Springer International Publishing.

Napi, N. M., Zaidan, A. A., Zaidan, B. B., Albahri, O. S., Alsalem, M. A., & Albahri, A. S. (2019). Medical emergency triage and patient propitiation in a telemedicine environment: a systematic review. *Health and Technology, 9*, 679-700.

Panch, T., Mattie, H., & Celi, L. A. (2019). The "inconvenient truth" about AI in healthcare. *NPJ digital medicine, 2*(1), 77.

Patel, S. (2023) *Chatbot for Healthcare: Key Use Cases & Benefits, REVE Chat.* Available at: https://www.revechat.com/blog/chatbot-for-healthcare/ (Accessed: 17 August 2023).

Patient Point (2023) *Patientpoint, PatientPoint.* Available at: https://www.patientpoint.com/ (Accessed: 11 July 2023).

Phillips, A. (2019). Effective approaches to health promotion in nursing practice. *Nursing Standard.*

Pianykh, O. S., Langs, G., Dewey, M., Enzmann, D. R., Herold, C. J., Schoenberg, S. O., & Brink, J. A. (2020). Continuous learning AI in radiology: implementation principles and early applications. *Radiology, 297*(1), 6-14.

ProPublica (2020) *Black women dying in pregnancy and childbirth at alarming rates, Giving Compass.* Available at: https://givingcompass.org/article/embedded-racial-inequities-in-delivery-rooms-and-beyond (Accessed: 17 July 2023).

Proskurnina, N. V., Shtal, T. V., Slavuta, O. I., Serogina, D. O., & Bohuslavskyi, V. V. (2021). Omnichannel Strategy of digital transformation of retail trade enterprise: From concept to implementation. *Studies of Applied Economics, 39*(6).

Purba, J. H. V., Ratodi, M., Mulyana, M., Wahyoedi, S., Andriana, R., Shankar, K., & Nguyen, P. T. (2019). Prediction model in medical science and health care. *Prediction Model in Medical Science and Health Care*, *8*(6S3).

Rama, A. (2019). National Health Expenditures, 2019: Steady spending growth despite increases in personal health care expenditures in advance of the pandemic. *AMA Policy Research Perspective.*

Rayan, N. (2019, December). Framework for analysis and detection of fraud in health insurance. In *2019 IEEE 6th International Conference on Cloud Computing and Intelligence Systems (CCIS)* (pp. 47-56). IEEE.

Reddy, S., Allan, S., Coghlan, S., & Cooper, P. (2020). A governance model for the application of AI in health care. *Journal of the American Medical Informatics Association*, *27*(3), 491-497.

Rodziewicz, T. L., & Hipskind, J. E. (2020). Medical error prevention. *StatPearls. Treasure Island (FL): StatPearls Publishing.*

Rosenbaum (2019) *New Medical Malpractice statistics by State, Rosenbaum.* Available at: https://www.rosenbaumfirm.com/medical-malpractice-statistics.html (Accessed: 17 July 2023).

Schacht, K., Furst, W., Jimbo, M., & Chavey, W. E. (2022). A malpractice claims study of a family medicine department: a 20-year review. *The Journal of the American Board of Family Medicine*, *35*(2), 380-386.

Secinaro, S., Calandra, D., Secinaro, A., Muthurangu, V., & Biancone, P. (2021). The role of artificial intelligence in healthcare: a structured literature review. *BMC medical informatics and decision making*, *21*, 1-23.

Shaheen, M. Y. (2021). Applications of Artificial Intelligence (AI) in healthcare: A review. *ScienceOpen Preprints*.

Singh, P. (2023) *How does an Omnichannel Marketing Benefit The Pharma Industry?*, *REVE Chat*. Available at: https://www.revechat.com/blog/omnichannel-pharma/ (Accessed: 17 August 2023).

Soroya, S. H., Farooq, A., Mahmood, K., Isoaho, J., & Zara, S. E. (2021). From information seeking to information avoidance: Understanding the health information behavior during a global health crisis. *Information processing & management*, *58*(2), 102440.

Stone, J. L., & Hoffman, G. (2010). *Medicare hospital readmissions: Issues, policy options and*

PPACA (pp. 1-37). Washington, DC: Congressional Research Service.

Strickland, E. (2019). IBM Watson, heal thyself: How IBM overpromised and underdelivered on AI health care. *IEEE Spectrum*, *56*(4), 24-31.

Sun, H., Xiao, J., Zhu, W., He, Y., Zhang, S., Xu, X., ... & Xie, G. (2020). Medical knowledge graph to enhance fraud, waste, and abuse detection on claim data: model development and performance evaluation. *JMIR Medical Informatics*, *8*(7), e17653.

Surkunte, A. (2022) *Technology innovation US Healthcare and health reforms*, *RSS*. Available at: https://www.magazine.medicaltourism.com/article/technology-innovation-us-healthcare-and-health-reforms (Accessed: 26 July 2023).

Tariq, M. I., Tayyaba, S., Ashraf, M. W., & Balas, V. E. (2020). Deep learning techniques for optimizing medical big data. In *Deep Learning Techniques for Biomedical and Health Informatics* (pp. 187-211). Academic Press.

Umoke, M., Umoke, P. C. I., Nwimo, I. O., Nwalieji, C. A., Onwe, R. N., Emmanuel Ifeanyi, N., & Samson Olaoluwa, A. (2020). Patients' satisfaction with quality of care in general hospitals in Ebonyi State, Nigeria, using SERVQUAL theory. *SAGE open medicine, 8,* 2050312120945129.

Van Calster, B., Wynants, L., Timmerman, D., Steyerberg, E. W., & Collins, G. S. (2019). Predictive analytics in health care: how can we know it works?. *Journal of the American Medical Informatics Association, 26*(12), 1651-1654.

Vega, R. J., & Kizer, K. W. (2020). VHA's innovation ecosystem: Operationalizing innovation in health care. *NEJM Catalyst Innovations in Care Delivery, 1*(6).

Viz.ai (2023) *Home, Viz.ai, the Proven AI-Powered Care Coordination Platform.* Available at: https://www.viz.ai/ (Accessed: 11 July 2023).

Wen, A., Fu, S., Moon, S., El Wazir, M., Rosenbaum, A., Kaggal, V. C., ... & Fan, J. (2019). Desiderata for delivering NLP to accelerate healthcare AI advancement and a Mayo Clinic NLP-as-a-service implementation. *NPJ digital medicine, 2*(1), 130.

Willink, S. (2021) *The UK's new approach to regulating artificial intelligence in Healthcare, Ideagen.* Available at: https://www.ideagen.com/thought-leadership/blog/the-uk-s-new-approach-to-regulating-artificial-intelligence-in-healthcare (Accessed: 10 July 2023).

Wurcel, V., Cicchetti, A., Garrison, L., Kip, M. M., Koffijberg, H., Kolbe, A., ... & Zamora, B. (2019). The value of diagnostic information in personalised healthcare: a comprehensive concept to facilitate bringing this technology into healthcare systems. *Public health genomics*, *22*(1-2), 8-15.

Xia, H., An, W., Li, J., & Zhang, Z. J. (2022). Outlier knowledge management for extreme public health events: Understanding public opinions about COVID-19 based on microblog data. *Socio-Economic Planning Sciences*, *80*, 100941.

Yaqoob, I., Salah, K., Jayaraman, R., & Al-Hammadi, Y. (2021). Blockchain for healthcare data management: opportunities, challenges, and future recommendations. *Neural Computing and Applications*, 1-16.

Zhou, Y., Xiang, S., Yang, F., & Lu, X. (2022). Targeting gatekeeper mutations for kinase drug discovery. *Journal of Medicinal Chemistry*, *65*(23), 15540-15558.

Glossary

American Institute of Medicine: It is an institute that is designed to provide leadership and educational training to aspirant medical practitioners and also involves itself in regulations of medical sciences and management.

Antidepressant Drugs: The antidepressants are used to treat depressive disorders, anxiety, pain and addiction. It involves the use of selective serotonin reuptake inhibitors, citalopram, fluvoxamine etc.

Artificial Intelligence: It is the intelligence of machine system through software to make decisions, and it marginalizes the requirement of human integration to operate systems.

Augmented Reality: It is the interaction of real-word with digitally generated content. The content incorporates visuals, auditory, and multiple sensory modalities.

Clinical Decision System: It is a system readily incorporated in health IT that assists clinician and practitioners with person-specific decision making and information to optimize quality of healthcare.

Convolution Neural Network: It is a neural network system dependent on feed-forward mechanism that self-engineers itself via filters of optimization. Regularized weights are assigned to prevent vanishing gradients and exploring gradients to improve the efficiency of neural imaging.

Deep Learning: It is a broader terminology used for machine learning. It uses multiple layer of analysis in the network for better assessment and result generation of the task assigned.

Digital Clock and Recall: It is a three-part test used for screening early dementia including possibilities of Alzheimer disease. It involves drawing a clock by hand from the patient with a specific time

Electronic Health Record: It is a digitally stores data on patient history and their associated diseases to assist in decision making of practitioners.

Fraud, Waste and Abuse detection and prevention: It is the process to optimize the usage of key health institution resources that may include material as well as medicine to practice resource optimality within health settings.

Gross Domestic Product: It is the monetary measure of collective market value that is within an economy or a region.

Health Insurance Portability and Accountability Act: It is a health insurance act under 104th United States Act of

Congress that is focused on ensuring efficient and affordable healthcare for patients.

Human Resource Information System: It is an information system that is designed to optimize workforce performance and accountability to ensure betterment in organizational performance. It is a digitally controlled software which offers management of workforce efficiently.

Information Technology: It is the use of machines to create, process, store, and exchange data including key information based on user requirement digitally.

Machine Learning: It is the self-generated algorithms by machines to solve an assigned problem using existing data set and humanized solutions that were incorporated in the past to train the existing and automated model.

Medical Malpractice: It is defined by medical practitioners' inability to abide by the code of conduct in medicine. It also involves negligent, illegal and improper behavior of practitioners.

Natural Language Processing: It is the application used to analyze speech and synthesize the components of human speech to computer technologies that assists in incorporation of technology.

Neural Networks: It is a method that is inhibited into a computer system to perform task and perform data in a method that is also used by human.

Patient Protection and Affordable Care Act: Also known as 'Obamacare', it is an act for the US citizens that ensures affordable and quality healthcare for their citizens.

Support Vector Machine: It is a sub-category of machine learning process that analyzes the network using regression analysis to optimize the effectiveness of its finding. It is used in healthcare and neural imaging for enhanced effectiveness.

Technology Acceptance Model: It is a theory based on information systems that revolves around the users' ability to understand technology. Behavioral intention is a key component of technology acceptance model.

www.ingramcontent.com/pod-product-compliance
Lightning Source LLC
Chambersburg PA
CBHW062332290526
45794CB00005B/2004